Maraña

Maraña

War and Disease in the Jungles of Colombia

LINA PINTO-GARCÍA

The University of Chicago Press
Chicago and London

The University of Chicago Press, Chicago 60637
The University of Chicago Press, Ltd., London

Published 2025
Printed in the United States of America

34 33 32 31 30 29 28 27 26 25   1 2 3 4 5

ISBN-13: 978-0-226-83932-5 (cloth)
ISBN-13: 978-0-226-83934-9 (paper)
ISBN-13: 978-0-226-83933-2 (e-book)
DOI: https://doi.org/10.7208/chicago/9780226839332.001.0001

Library of Congress Cataloging-in-Publication Data

Names: Pinto-García, Lina, author.
Title: Maraña : war and disease in the jungles of Colombia / Lina Pinto-García.
Description: Chicago : The University of Chicago Press, 2025. |
Includes bibliographical references and index.
Identifiers: LCCN 2024037630 | ISBN 9780226839325 (cloth) |
ISBN 9780226839349 (paperback) | ISBN 9780226839332 (ebook)
Subjects: LCSH: Leishmaniasis, Cutaneous. | Political violence—Colombia. |
War—Medical aspects.
Classification: LCC RL764.C8 P56 2025 | DDC 616.9/364—dc23/eng/20241101
LC record available at https://lccn.loc.gov/2024037630

♾ This paper meets the requirements of ANSI/NISO Z39.48-1992 (Permanence of Paper).

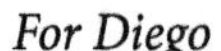

For Diego

Contents

Note on Terminology

Spanish is the language of my fieldwork and most of the documentary sources in this book. It is therefore necessary to clarify some of the terminology used in the following pages. It should also be noted that quotations from texts originally written in Spanish are my English translations.

Leishmaniasis

The field of biomedicine describes two main forms of leishmaniasis: cutaneous and visceral. The term *leishmaniases* is often used to refer to both forms. Unless otherwise indicated, I use *leishmaniasis* to refer to cutaneous leishmaniasis, the disease with which this book is concerned.

Jungle, Forest, and *Selva*

In Colombia, people generally use the Spanish word *selva* to refer to the lush vegetation ecologies where both war and cutaneous leishmaniasis proliferate. *Selva* is commonly translated into English as "jungle." However, academic works that have addressed the complex and many-sided relationship between this environment and the Colombian armed conflict have retained the use of *selva* or preferred the word *forest* to distance themselves from the colonial legacy attached to the term *jungle* (Lyons 2020; Ruiz-Serna 2023). They argue that *jungle* exoticizes and reinforces the idea that forests belong to the north while jungles belong to the south. Lyons (2020, 8) finds problematic the use of *forest*, as it evokes monocultures of timber trees, which renders invisible the exuberant biodiversity underlying the messy, relational, and metamorphic nature of *selva*.

Yet I say that *selva* cannot be absolved from these colonial or reductionist traps. As works by Rodríguez (1997), Serje (2005), and Ospina (2014) point out, the unfinished colonial history of what is present-day Colombia has time and again relied on the word *selva* to refer to savage territories that harbor untapped riches and indomitable violence. This connotation is especially present in the term *sylvatic*, etymologically derived from *selva*, which is used in epidemiology to define the transmission cycle of diseases such as cutaneous leishmaniasis. As Duarte da Silva (2023) explains, sylvatic denotes uninhabited and wild spaces in need of civilization, an idea that was at the heart of European colonial expansion in the Americas, Asia, Africa, and Oceania.

I return to this topic in the introduction of this book. For the moment, let me clarify that my interchangeable use of the words *jungle*, *forest*, and *rainforest* is not naive to this debate but rather an English-reader-friendly way to refer to spaces where all kinds of species, entities, and beings relate to each other and become deeply entangled with human and more-than-human phenomena that develop within them, like war and leishmaniasis. While admittedly problematic, neither the colloquial use of the word *selva* nor its untranslated use in English texts can escape those same problems.

Soldier and Army

In this book, if not specified otherwise, the word *soldier(s)* always refers to members of the Colombian state Army and the word *Army*, with a capital letter, always refers to the Colombian state Army.

FARC

Among the actors I mention most often in this book are the members of the now-dissolved guerrilla organization Revolutionary Armed Forces of Colombia–People's Army (Fuerzas Armadas Revolucionarias de Colombia–Ejército del Pueblo). To refer to this guerrilla group, I use the acronym FARC rather than the official acronym FARC-EP because this is how people in Colombia commonly refer to this organization.

Paramilitaries

Alongside the leftist guerrillas and the state Army, right-wing paramilitary groups are the third major player in the Colombian armed conflict. Among the paramilitaries, the United Self-Defenders of Colombia (Autodefensas Unidas de Colombia; AUC), formed in 1997, was the largest group. According to a major historical memory report published in 2013, paramilitaries have been the cruelest and bloodiest armed actors carrying out the major and most atrocious massacres, targeted killings, and enforced disappearances of the Colombian armed conflict, on many occasions with support and collaboration from the state (CNMH 2013). Despite the controversial demobilization of the AUC that took place between 2003 and 2006, the paramilitary movement was not dismantled. Although the state has often claimed that paramilitaries do not exist as they used to, it uses the terms *bandas criminales* (criminal gangs), or *bacrim*, to name the paramilitary structures that still operate today (Valencia and Montoya 2016). Civil society organizations have called these groups *neoparamilitaries, third generation of paramilitaries, heirs of the paramilitaries*, or simply *paramilitaries* (Masse 2011). Throughout this book, I use the term *paramilitaries.*

War Names

Names set in single quotation marks are *nombres de guerra* (war names) chosen by members of guerrilla groups or given to them when they join guerrilla organizations.

Departamentos

Colombia is politically and administratively divided into thirty-seven territorial divisions made up of thirty-two *departamentos* and five districts. Throughout this book, I use the Spanish word *departamento(s).* Boyacá, Guaviare, Tolima, Caquetá, and Putumayo are some of the *departamentos* I mention frequently. I also refer several times to the government entities responsible for health at the departmental level—the Departmental Health Secretariats.

Public Force

In Colombia, the term *Fuerza Pública* (Public Force) encompasses both the military forces (Army, Navy, and Air Force) and the National Police.

Introduction

Andrea González[1] spent two years traveling on board helicopters of the Colombian Army—at least once a week between 2006 and 2008. These helicopters were routinely used to shuttle soldiers in and out of combat zones; rescue the wounded; and supply food, ammunition, and other provisions to troops scattered in densely forested areas of the Amazon region. However, Andrea was involved in a very different operation—a scientific one. As a university researcher with a background in microbiology, she was coordinating a clinical trial that recruited military participants to investigate biomedical therapies against cutaneous leishmaniasis.

The characteristic sign of this disease is a rounded, hollowed-out, and raw skin sore that forms after a sandfly bites and transmits microscopic *Leishmania* parasites to a person. The standard treatment used to heal these ulcers in Colombia is a drug with the brand name Glucantime. The clinical trial led by Andrea sought to compare this pharmaceutical with two other therapies. To do so, the trial protocol prescribed two additional follow-ups to be conducted with the participants three and six months after the end of the treatment. Andrea and her colleagues had to devise a plan for her to execute the follow-up treatment visits even though her trial soldier-patients had already returned to the front lines of combat in the jungle. It was decided that she would join routine military helicopter operations to the tropical forest zones in order to access her military patients and document the effect that these experimental antileishmanial therapies had on a trial group of 437 soldiers.

From the helicopter, the thickly meshed canopy of trees resembled a giant green and velvety carpet stretching out on the horizon. Once on the ground, however, this seemingly homogeneous living mass took on a very different appearance. Composed of an extraordinary diversity of plants that compete for every available corner and ray of sunlight, the rainforest shows itself as an intricate tangle of multiple forms and textures, colored by shadows and the most varied palette of humid greens, blues, and browns. For over five decades, this densely forested tropical environment has served as the main stage for Colombia's armed conflict—*el conflicto armado*, one of the longest and most violent wars in Latin American history.

Besides demarcating the zones of conflict, the ecological borders of the tropical jungle also delimit the spaces of existence for minute sandflies that transmit leishmaniasis. In this lush setting, rock crevices, nests, the undersides of leaves, animal burrows, and the uneven surfaces of tree trunks offer humid and dark dwellings for these insects to spend most of the day in hiding. At twilight, however, female sandflies become particularly active, seeking mammals to bite and obtain the blood they need to develop their eggs. Opossums, armadillos, sloths, anteaters, bats, wild rats, porcupines, pumas, and jaguars are attractive sources of blood for these insects—and so are two-legged mammals, many of them armed and dressed in camouflage. To the sandflies, these beings simply represent yet another source of nourishment, one that became particularly abundant and available with the armed conflict. As a result, Army soldiers, guerrillas, and paramilitaries constitute the populations most affected by leishmaniasis in Colombia.

As long as the helicopter was not ambushed from below, it would land, permitting its onboard military personnel and Andrea to hop off in order to fulfill their respective assigned missions. Fearing a sudden guerrilla attack, military members loaded and unloaded provisions and people from the aircraft with feverish haste. Concurrently, as the rotating helicopter blades roared beside her, Andrea quickly assessed and documented the healing progress of each of the soldiers who were participants in her trial. Andrea recounted her experience to me ten years later in her university office, far away from the Amazon and the daily tensions of war. "I saw many young men without legs, even a twenty-two-year-old soldier whose face had been completely blown up by a land mine, eyes included; it was absolutely sad and horrifying," she told me. Andrea kept stressing how different and impressive it was to be in the forested and remote areas of the country, confronting the war face-to-face. In her opinion, her experience was in sharp contrast to that of most Colombians in the main cities who had become used to watching the events of the war on television. "It was a titanic job, a suicide job. I even had to do it on Christmas Day. It was very difficult to coordinate all this with the Army commanders. But that work was great. I loved it!" she said. I asked her whether she might have had the same sort of experience if she had been doing research on a disease other than leishmaniasis. "No, it's very unlikely, it's very unlikely," she answered.

Such stories never made it into the scientific articles that Andrea and her colleagues published on the clinical trial, and they remain undocumented to this day. Leishmaniasis researchers do not tend to divulge their experiences on the ground, except as anecdotes that might informally arise as hallway conversation or during the coffee breaks at scientific conferences. As such, they are not part of the "official" accounts about leishmaniasis found in scientific journals or public health documents. Scenes like these remain marginal, unfamiliar, and, for the most part, unknown to the (scientific) world. Thus, people wearing immaculate lab coats and latex gloves in quiet and aseptic rooms, illuminated with cold white lamps still make up the iconic image—but not necessarily the reality—that is associated with leishmaniasis-related biomedical research and clinical studies in Colombia.

Yet this skin vector-borne disease is deeply intertwined with the complex armed conflict the country has experienced for decades. When you examine Colombian leishmaniasis closely, as I have, you will inevitably encounter all sorts of actors, objects, violences, inequities, knowledges, and imaginaries engendered, shaped, connected, and kept alive by war. I would have, as Andrea implied, been significantly less likely to uncover the picture that I present in the following pages had my focus been on a disease other than leishmaniasis.

Among those who have heard about leishmaniasis in Colombia, this disease—like no other—is often stigmatized as "the guerrilla disease" or "the subversive disease" (see, for instance, Molano Bravo 2005b; Emanuelsson 2012). Although leishmaniasis does not affect only guerrilla members, the misconception that it is solely a guerrilla illness has deeply infused certain imaginaries with gruesome, even deadly consequences for some people in rural areas. Significantly, this stigmatization has been reinforced by the fact that the state has established restrictive control on access to antileishmanial medications, a measure that is locally interpreted as a warfare strategy aimed to disadvantage insurgent groups living in close relationships with the forested ecologies and sandflies that inhabit them.

* * *

This book explores the intricate entanglements of cutaneous leishmaniasis with the Colombian armed conflict. It provides deep insight into the ways in which war is capable of transforming social life and altering everyday and cultural practices, including those related to public health, medical practice, biomedical research, and the political economy and regulation of pharmaceuticals. As such, domains that are typically considered peaceful and unrelated to war appear here as directly implicated in a multidimensional web of intentional and unintentional violence. The people who populate these pages are the ones you would expect in any account of the Colombian war: soldiers, guerrillas, paramilitaries, and civilians caught up in all sorts of tangible and symbolic cross fires. But other, less usual actors are also central to this story: scientists, health care workers, public health officials, microscopic parasites, sandflies, and the forested ecologies in which leishmaniasis develops.

This ethnographic exploration of the social world of leishmaniasis in the context of the Colombian armed conflict builds a more complex understanding of the ontologies of both this disease and the war. It subverts the nature/culture dichotomy by showing how leishmaniasis constitutes a pathological dimension of the armed conflict involving multiple kinds of nonhuman entities. In this way, this book challenges the definition of war as a purely human phenomenon. Also, by highlighting the prominent role played by the armed conflict in the epidemiology and experience of leishmaniasis, this work destabilizes the Pasteurian idea that an infectious disease is defined by the pathogen that causes it. Here, leishmaniasis does not appear as something ontologically natural but as a phenomenon inseparable from culture and the violence that humans bring about amid political and social conflict.

My argument is that Colombian leishmaniasis cannot be understood as an isolated disease, disconnected from the specifics of the Colombian armed conflict. This disease and the war are not merely linked; they are also entangled with each other through discourses, rationales, technologies, and practices produced by the state, medicine, biomedical research, and the armed conflict itself. As such, this interaction implies much more than a circumstantial and unfortunate encounter between leishmaniasis-transmitting sandflies and combatants in the jungle. This work shows the critical centrality of the conflict for the experience of leishmaniasis in Colombia, which renders incomplete any account of this disease that does not take into serious consideration the various ramifications and localized expressions of the war. Put differently, leishmaniasis has been socially, discursively, and materially constructed as *a disease of the war* with the crucial participation of public health, medicine, and especially pharmaceutical drugs. The case of Colombian leishmaniasis instantiates how a violent context produces a violent technoscience that, in turn, produces knowledge and resources that contribute to maintaining violence within society.

I have chosen to represent the intricate association between this disease and the Colombian armed conflict as an intertwined *maraña*. *Maraña* is a Spanish word that means "tangle," but it is also commonly used in Colombia to refer to the tropical jungle. I was reminded of this by several soldiers affected by leishmaniasis with whom I had the opportunity and privilege to talk during my many months of fieldwork. *Maraña* refers to the thickness of the rainforest, to its entangled and intertwined greenery, to braided lianas and dense foliage that make any trek through it challenging. When soldiers enter this forested landscape, they talk about *enmarañarse* (getting tangled up), sneaking into the vegetation, becoming part of the *maraña*, getting so entwined with it, and submitting to its vicissitudes that *desenmarañarse* (disentangling oneself) turns into a complicated task. *Maraña* is a conceptual resource that I have collected from the voices of my research participants to explain the kind of human and more-than-human contingencies, relationships, and moving elements that give rise to leishmaniasis within biodiverse spaces historically affected by the war. Through the *maraña*, I metaphorically describe the relationship between leishmaniasis and the conflict as a messy arrangement of lianas that hold these two phenomena together in multiple and interconnected ways. As a concept, *maraña* also stresses that although leishmaniasis and conflict have become *enmarañados* (tangled up)—which makes it fundamentally impossible to make sense of this disease if the war is overlooked or downplayed—they can also become *desenmarañados* (disentangled). Since their attachments are relational and not inherent to them, leishmaniasis and war can—and should—constitute a different type of relationship for those who have historically lived with both the disease and the conflict. Their disentanglement starts with careful analysis of the complex interplay between war and disease in order to make visible the violences underpinning the current social order that must be addressed—and repaired.

In biomedical and public health discourses, the armed conflict is commonly described as a "social determinant" of leishmaniasis in Colombia (see, for instance, INS and ONS 2017). However, the interactions between these two phenomena have remained only superficially explored and documented, and "conflict" tends to be assumed as a reified notion—often a metric—which makes it very hard to actually understand how the complex and variable nature of armed violence has contributed to disease and ill health. Furthermore, the understanding of conflict as a determinant factor of leishmaniasis reduces the relationship to a unidirectional arrow that obscures the ways in which leishmaniasis, and the state's strategy to biomedically address this disease, may also be a cause of violence and further deterioration of human health. This book draws attention to the armed conflict and the ways in which it has crucially shaped the morbidity and epidemiology of leishmaniasis in Colombia. Similarly, it documents how leishmaniasis in turn has shaped the course of the armed conflict in distinctive ways. It does due diligence to the relationship between leishmaniasis and war by qualifying, complicating, and enriching this association with ethnographic content and visceral experiences that demonstrate their undeniable and persistent *enmarañamiento* in the Colombian context.

Developing a deeper understanding of the interplay of conflict and leishmaniasis seems particularly relevant at a time when Colombia is going through a challenging peace-building process after the 2016 signing of a peace agreement between the state and the largest and oldest guerrilla organization in the Americas—the FARC. Yet this work has relevance for other territories affected by similar disease "remnants" of war (Redfield and Rackley 2009). It is at this critical turning point in Colombian history that a study of the tightly coupled association between leishmaniasis and the armed conflict can contribute to understanding the role that science, medicine, and pharmaceutical technologies have played in the inescapable, pervasive, and corrosive phenomenon of war. Crucially, it can also contribute to envisioning how health care and biomedical research can be transformed and repurposed toward social justice efforts and the aspirations of overcoming violence in Colombia and elsewhere. Moreover, the analysis I provide here offers key reflections on how to better frame and address health problems and inequalities that affect populations in areas where war has disrupted life for decades.

By putting the focus on leishmaniasis, I show how and why this disease has become a *patología de la patria* (homeland pathology) in war-ridden Colombia—that is, a disease encapsulating not only violent years of social and armed conflict but also the state's conception of its enemies, rural populations and spaces, development and progress, and legitimate ways of waging war. For historians Hochman, Di Liscia, and Palmer (2012, 13–27), *homeland pathologies* are scientific constructions of diseases that, in specific moments of Latin American modern history, have served to delimit spaces and identify certain populations for their further—but conditioned—incorporation into nation-building projects. Homeland pathologies indicate time-space particularities that, through the use of medical labels, constitute, demarcate, and bring to the fore populations embodying aspects of the nation perceived as negative, which need to be addressed through medical-scientific and public health strategies. These diseases do not necessarily have to be epidemiologically problematized as serious health issues. Instead, their configuration as *homeland pathologies* and their elevation as national concerns depend on contingent factors capable of establishing associations and affinities between individuals and spaces, their imbrication with larger national problems and projects, and biomedical intervention as a state duty.

As a homeland pathology in contemporary Colombia, leishmaniasis is an illness that condenses many of the social dynamics and patterns characterizing a period of national history marked by the armed conflict. This disease works as an entry point to explore how a disease and its associated technologies, biomedical understandings, and practices can be shaped, instrumentalized, and resignified to produce violence, stigmatization, and exclusion in a context of conflict. Thus, this book is an example of how ethnographic approaches rooted in science and technology studies (STS) and critical medical anthropology can contribute to the unveiling—and eventual disruption—of the role of pharmaceuticals and biomedical epistemologies, spaces, and practices in the production of unanticipated battlefields and repertoires of violence that are otherwise rarely recognized as such.

In this work, I often speak of *Colombian leishmaniasis*. My use of this terminology does not correspond in any way to the nomenclature used by scientists or to a specific species of the *Leishmania* parasite. When I speak of Colombian leishmaniasis, I am drawing on Margaret Lock's conceptualization of *local biologies* to point at the convergence between biological and social elements that constitute leishmaniasis in Colombia. I refer to this disease as a *biosocial* phenomenon that originates in a particular time and space (Lock and Nguyen 2010). I do this as a way of problematizing the main working assumption of biomedicine: that all bodies are biologically the same, independently from where they are geographically, politically, and historically located (Lock 1995). In contrast, the *Colombian leishmaniasis* terminology underscores that this disease is the result of particular cultural and historical trajectories in which the armed conflict remains deeply implicated in the local experience and knowledge of leishmaniasis.

Maraña and Disentanglement

My understanding of the *maraña* formed by leishmaniasis and the war departs from predominant anthropocentric approaches that make sense of violence and armed conflicts as quintessentially human-made phenomena, involving exclusively human victims, perpetrators, and witnesses. Instead, I understand war as the product of a heterogeneous collective of living and nonliving entities, "where nature and culture are being refigured, where humans and nonhumans are being remade by discourses and material practices" (Kosek 2010, 653). Thus *maraña* is a material-semiotic reworking of the armed conflict (Law 2008). It expands on the efforts of other scholars who consider the intricate socioecological relationships between humans and nonhumans as crucial agents in shaping history, waging war, and producing violence (De León 2015; Pugliese 2020; Ruiz-Serna 2023; Ruiz-Serna and Ojeda 2023).[2] As such, *maraña* involves a relational approach to the understanding of war that builds on, but also goes beyond the ordinary limits of, both the humanist perspective on the Colombian armed conflict and the anthropocentric frame of peace-building processes.

Drawing on Karen Barad's work, Alex Nading (2014) has heavily relied on the notion of *entanglement* to illustrate the intricate, complex, and unbreakable connections between the humans and nonhumans that make up dengue in Nicaragua. In physics, two particles are said to be "entangled" when, although being separated in space, they *cannot* be independently described because the state of one is connected and dependent on the state of the other. For Nading, *entanglement* indexes indestructible human-nonhuman relationships whose subtraction would render incomplete any understanding of dengue. Although *entanglement* is often translated into Spanish as *enmarañamiento*, I want to indicate in what ways this notion resembles and differs from the concept of *maraña* in this book.

While *entanglement* and *maraña* have the relational connotation in common, I see *maraña* as the result of the processes of *enmarañamiento* and the actions of *enmarañar* (tangling up) that, unlike entanglement, can be undone by unraveling—at least partially—that which holds its elements together. Even though my inquiry does rely on *entanglement*'s relational emphasis to highlight the impossibility of making sense of leishmaniasis without factoring in the war, and also to describe how and why leishmaniasis and the armed conflict have established complex links to each other with the constant implication of nonhumans, I refrain from seeing these two as inseparable phenomena. I contend that leishmaniasis and the armed conflict *can* break the ties that have connected them in wartime and that they *should* constitute another type of relationship—a *disentangled* one—in times of peace. In other words, if the *enmarañamiento* of war and leishmaniasis is not inevitable, their disentanglement should be possible. Moreover, by emphasizing the "conditions of pathogenic possibility" that converge in a specific time and space (H. Brown and Kelly 2014, 282), *maraña* denotes a strong sense of place that *entanglement* fails to convey. As such, *maraña* forces us to always think with—and never without—the ecological, material, and social conditions that enable leishmaniasis development in historically and spatially situated ways (Peluso and Watts 2001).

If I consider that the armed conflict and leishmaniasis can be disentangled, it is not because I understand the separation between the social world and leishmaniasis as something possible. In tune with long-standing findings in STS and medical anthropology, diseases, as any other representation of nature constructed through scientific practices and discourses, always embed and are embedded in particular social arrangements, values, and historical trajectories (Latour 1993; Lock 1995). Thus, to *desenmarañar* (disentangle) war and leishmaniasis in Colombia involves reconstructing the links holding these phenomena together through processes guided by the goals and principles of peace building and social justice (Woodhouse et al. 2002). Disentanglement, then, is a normative stance that underscores the need to produce *other* attachments between leishmaniasis and society through *different* scientific programs, technological designs, health care practices, regulations, and social and cultural processes capable of challenging violence, suffering, and inequality.

The possibility for *disentanglement*, which I suggest is partially attainable if we think with the *maraña*, also draws on the work of Eva Haifa Giraud (2019). Recognizing the ethical, political, and material need to understand that nature and culture are not mutually exclusive ontological categories, her work is in line with a large body of STS scholarship that strives to unsettle anthropocentric and binary worldviews by insisting that the human condition depends on and is constituted by complex and entangled relationships with nonhumans (Haraway 2003; Strathern 1980). However, Giraud sustains that this "irreducible complexity . . . can prove paralyzing and disperse responsibilities in ways that undermine political action" (2019, 2). Giraud explores the possibility of political action to build more ethical and livable futures despite and amid entangled complexities. She proposes the adoption of an *ethics of exclusion*, which pays attention to those relationships, practices, and more-than-human arrangements "that are *foreclosed* when other entangled realities are materialized" (2019, 2). In other words, it is not enough to give meaning to the world by shedding light on existing and problematic entanglements between human and nonhuman entities. It is necessary to think about the reverse side of entanglement, that is, the exclusions built into the entanglements of the present to create the alternative relationships that make up the futures we hope to live in.

Considering the need for disentanglement of the *maraña* formed by leishmaniasis and the Colombian armed conflict, throughout this work I draw attention to some of the relationships and practices that would have to be excluded in order for another type of associations to emerge and materialize. Thus, the concept of *maraña* highlights the convoluted and messy relationships holding together leishmaniasis and war in Colombia, but also the hopeful possibility of their *desenmarañamiento* (disentanglement). *Desenmarañamiento* forces us to think creatively beyond simple "solutions" that, by reducing a highly complex problem to a quick technological fix (e.g., developing a magic-bullet drug or vaccine), fail to address the roots of the problem, offer at best a palliative remedy, and often create additional drawbacks. Thinking in terms of disentanglement means recognizing that technology can be part of the solution, but it is not *the* solution to the range of problems posed by the *maraña* formed by war and disease. It is about working across disciplines to develop various interventions of a sociotechnical and cultural nature—what Linda Layne (2000) calls social-technical and cultural fixes—to address the wide range of problems enmeshed in the *maraña*.

Leishmaniasis as a Biomedical Category with Occupational Implications

In the biomedical world, the word *leishmaniasis* refers to a broad spectrum of illnesses that have been grouped into two major—and very different—forms of the disease: cutaneous leishmaniasis and visceral leishmaniasis. Visceral leishmaniasis, also known by the Hindi term *kala-azar*, affects the internal organs of the body and is generally fatal if left untreated. Cutaneous leishmaniasis—the disease this book is concerned with—is neither deadly nor contagious and only affects the skin. Scientists have described more than twenty parasites of the *Leishmania* type as causative agents of leishmaniasis. From a biomedical standpoint, these microscopic creatures are transmitted to mammals—humans included—through the bite of tiny female sandflies that feed on blood to develop their eggs. Of approximately eight hundred species of sandflies, entomologists consider at least ninety-eight of them vectors of leishmaniasis (WHO 2010).

In the case of cutaneous leishmaniasis, weeks or months after an infected female sandfly has bitten someone, a skin lesion develops, generally in the spot of the bite. It starts out like a tiny sore that keeps growing and forms an ulcer. The typical textbook leishmaniasis lesion is commonly described in daily medical practice as a *volcancito* (little volcano)—a circular sore with a raised edge and a reddish-pink crater that might suppurate or be covered with a scab (fig. I.1). However, ulcers can have all sorts of shapes and sizes. Most are painless and grow slowly, and several cases clear up spontaneously, without the need for treatment. In the Americas, this so-called spontaneous self-healing or self-resolving cutaneous leishmaniasis is estimated to occur in 6–26 percent of people and varies depending on the parasite species (Fernandes Cota et al. 2016). Therefore, cutaneous leishmaniasis tends to be considered a mostly benign disease, especially when compared to life-threatening visceral leishmaniasis. Nevertheless, a leishmaniasis skin lesion might cause pain, particularly when it gets secondarily infected with fungi or bacteria, which is sometimes accompanied by a swollen, festering, and smelly appearance. Also, having a sore that, as days go by, expands toward the sides and depth of the skin is not only disturbing and uncomfortable but also might trigger feelings of disgust of oneself and others. In some cases, leishmaniasis lesions develop into chronic ulcers that do not heal, can last for several years, and often do not respond to drugs (see Fernández et al. 2014).

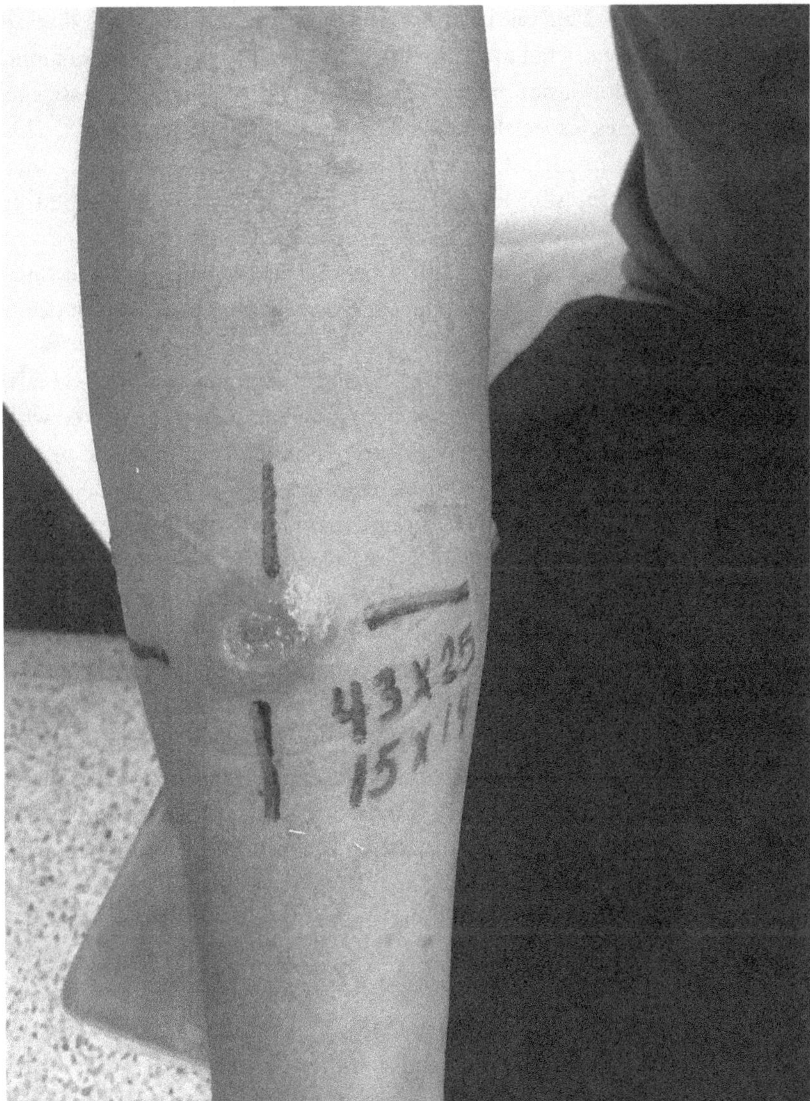

FIGURE I.1. Cutaneous leishmaniasis lesion on the right arm of a Colombian Army soldier. The lines drawn with a black marker are used to define and measure the boundaries of the lesion and to determine whether the lesion is shrinking as a result of drug treatment. Photo by Lina Pinto-García.

Although the much less frequently occurring diffuse and mucosal leishmaniasis are sometimes named as two additional forms of the disease, they are commonly understood as under- and overresponsive presentations of cutaneous leishmaniasis, respectively (Rojas et al. 2006). Diffuse leishmaniasis is characterized by multiple and widely disseminated lesions on the skin that do not form ulcers. Mucosal leishmaniasis is seen as a form of the disease that is exclusively restricted to the Americas, occurring when the *Leishmania* parasites from a skin lesion migrate through blood or lymphatic vessels to mucous membranes, especially those of the nose, mouth, and throat. This migration process, or metastasis, can take place either simultaneously with the appearance of the skin lesion or sometimes even years after the ulcer has healed. Mucosal leishmaniasis can sometimes result in mutilations and deformities of the nose, mouth, and throat, and in extreme cases, secondary bacterial overinfection of the upper respiratory tract can result in death (MinSalud and INS 2017).

The spectrum of leishmaniasis also includes asymptomatic individuals, that is, people who, despite having been bitten by sandflies and infected with *Leishmania* parasites, never develop ulcers. Although asymptomatic people are clinically unimportant and very hard to quantify, they are relevant in terms of public health because they can act as sources of infection for sandflies that can bite other people and make them sick (Rosales-Chilama et al. 2015). WorldLeish is the largest international conference on leishmaniasis, and in 2017 in Toledo, several scientists used the image of an iceberg to represent the place of asymptomatic patients in the current biomedical understanding of the disease. While the small and visible tip of the iceberg corresponded to the cases that are detectable to the eye in clinical practice, the large part—submerged, unseen, and understudied—represented the asymptomatic cases.

About 70–75 percent of the two hundred thousand annual cases of cutaneous leishmaniasis in the world are found in ten countries: Afghanistan, Iran, Syria, Algeria, Ethiopia, North Sudan, Costa Rica, Peru, Brazil, and Colombia. Taking into account the serious problem of underreporting in official public health surveillance data, it has been estimated that there are between 0.7 and 1.2 million cases of cutaneous leishmaniasis each year worldwide (Alvar et al. 2012). Although cutaneous leishmaniasis is widely distributed around the globe, generalizations and comparisons among regions of the world are not always easy or useful because the disease in its multiple forms develops and manifests differently, particularly from one side of the Atlantic Ocean to the other. Depending on the parasite and vector species, the ecological characteristics of the transmission sites, and the previous and current exposure of humans to the parasites, the manifestation of leishmaniasis varies broadly from one place to another (WHO 2010).

While there is a large gap in terms of scholarly works studying the social and political history of leishmaniasis,[3] some scientists have produced practitioner-centered histories about the people involved in the establishment of leishmaniasis as a medical category during the British occupation of India (Steverding 2017; Vincent 2017). These texts do not explicitly discuss but do implicitly reveal that leishmaniasis shares the same colonial and military patterns behind the scientific origin of other vector-borne diseases such as malaria and yellow fever (Espinosa 2009; Packard 2011; Quevedo V. et al. 2017). Significantly, concerns about kala-azar (visceral leishmaniasis) among the British became prominent in the late nineteenth century when tea plantation workers were highly affected by this disease in northeast India, resulting in a loss of revenue and profit for the British government (Dutta 2008). Although this disease's symptoms resembled those of malaria, patients did not respond to the quinine treatment. Thus, several researchers were appointed to investigate the etiology of the disease and determine whether it was just another bad form of malaria or perhaps something different. The scientific description of the association between *Leishmania* parasites and kala-azar in 1903 is attributed primarily to Lieutenant General William Leishman. He was a Scottish military physician who, after serving with the British Army in India, became part of the medical staff at the Royal Victoria Hospital in Netley, England. There, Leishman noticed some unknown parasites in smears taken postmortem from the spleen of a soldier who had been in Calcutta and published his observations in 1903. In the same year, Charles Donovan, an Irish doctor, member of the Indian Medical Service—the military medical service in British India—and professor at the Madras Medical College, reported the same sort of parasites in the spleens of both dead and living kala-azar patients (Dutta 2008). It was Ronald Ross—the same military doctor who received the 1902 Nobel Prize for identifying the pathogenic relationship among malaria, parasites, and mosquitoes—who acted as a liaison between Leishman and Donovan and who proposed that the new parasite should be called *Leishmania donovani* (Gibson 1983).

In 1904, Leishman associated this visceral leishmaniasis parasite with similar ones found in skin sores by American pathologist James Homer Wright. As Louis-Patrick Haraoui notes: "This was the first established link between clinical entities with very distinct symptomatology: usually benign skin lesions on the one hand, and severe, fatal involvement of the internal organs on the other" (2007, 62). Further descriptions of other *Leishmania* parasites causing either the deadly (visceral) or the nondeadly (cutaneous) forms of leishmaniasis followed. In the Americas, descriptions of cutaneous leishmaniasis that began appearing in 1909 changed what European tropical medicine centers involved in the colonial project considered established about leishmaniasis. In fact, the disease and its very diverse clinical manifestations became an important opportunity for exchange between South American and European specialists (Jogas Junior and Benchimol 2020). On the American continent, different *Leishmania* parasites causing cutaneous leishmaniasis started to be named in 1911. Many of them—*L. peruviana*, *L. braziliensis*, *L. guyanensis*, *L. amazonensis*, *L. panamensis*, *L. venezuelensis*, *L. mexicana*, *L. colombiensis*, and so on—were given scientific names that index their local and geographical particularities, as well as the broad diversity of parasites involved in leishmaniasis on the corresponding side of the Atlantic.[4] Similarly, the disease itself has also been historically named according to spatial and imperial references. Even today, in several parts of the world, cutaneous leishmaniasis is known by names that perpetuate and give primacy to colonial imaginaries attached to particular people and geographies, such as Aleppo evil, Baghdad boil, Delhi boil, and Oriental sore (see Bowker and Star 1999, 79–80).

Reminiscent of imperialism and the colonial origins of leishmaniasis as a biomedical category, scientists still use the New/Old World terminology to highlight epidemiological differences between the two world hemispheres. Cutaneous leishmaniasis on the American continent—what scientists refer to as "New World cutaneous leishmaniasis" or "American cutaneous leishmaniasis"—is predominantly related to jungle ecologies, not to the semi-arid or even desert conditions of cutaneous leishmaniasis transmission in other parts of the world. In fact, the term *sylvatic* is usually employed in epidemiology to describe the *Leishmania* parasite life and transmission cycles involving sandflies and nonhuman mammals amid the forested ecologies that characterize much of Colombia's rurality. *Sylvatic* implies wild, uninhabited, and sometimes even pristine forested spaces where the insect vector and the mammalian reservoir live and maintain *Leishmania* parasites independently from humans. Under this interpretation, the temporary irruption of humans into these jungle ecologies makes them vulnerable to leishmaniasis and turns them into "accidental hosts due to the vector's search for blood source" (Ferro et al. 2015, 1). As Matheus Duarte da Silva (2023) explains, framing spaces as wild and empty of humans through the use of the term *sylvatic* is deeply associated with a mindset rooted in European colonial expansion, which was particularly applied to the Amazon rainforest. Yet the description of cutaneous leishmaniasis in Colombia as a sylvatic disease is not restricted to the Amazon region but to forested, rural, and remote areas distributed nationwide. In fact, based on case reporting to the state, leishmaniasis is considered endemic throughout the country, except for the islands of San Andrés, the *departamento* of Atlántico, and the capital city, Bogotá (MinSalud and INS 2017).

On the American continent, cutaneous leishmaniasis has been primarily seen as an occupational disease affecting mostly men who enter or live in close contact with the jungle because of the economic activity they are involved in (Weigle et al. 1993; WHO 2010; Benchimol et al. 2019). In Central America, for instance, the disease is known as *úlcera del chiclero*, highlighting how it has predominantly affected workers who tap chicle (gum) trees. In Colombia, cutaneous leishmaniasis has been commonly regarded as a disease affecting men who are in contact with the jungle because of the work they do, especially combatants directly involved in the protracted armed conflict that has unfolded within this landscape. In recent years, however, those who study leishmaniasis in Colombia have noticed an increase in cases among women and children. They often attribute this to the fact that the transmission of the disease is no longer only sylvatic but also domestic and peridomestic, due to urbanization and deforestation processes (see, for instance, Rodríguez-Barraquer et al. 2008). This interpretation, however, overlooks the fact that women and minors are often part of nonstate armed groups or workers in economies considered illicit, such as the coca leaf cultivation and harvest. Nevertheless, the relationship between leishmaniasis and rural and forested ecologies continues to dominate the epidemiological understanding of the disease in the country.

The vast majority (95–98 percent) of all leishmaniasis cases in Colombia correspond to cutaneous leishmaniasis. In fact, Colombia has the second-highest number of cutaneous leishmaniasis cases after Brazil in the Americas. While visceral leishmaniasis also occurs in the country, this form of the disease accounts for less than 1.5 percent of all leishmaniasis cases and remains concentrated in two specific and well-characterized areas that are different from the jungle ecosystems where cutaneous leishmaniasis develops (INS 2017). Thus, when the term *leishmaniasis* is employed in Colombia without the words *visceral* or *mucosal* qualifying it, people are most certainly referring to cutaneous leishmaniasis. As I have done so far, I adopt the same usage throughout this book. Unless otherwise indicated, I use the word *leishmaniasis* to refer to cutaneous leishmaniasis, the disease that is strongly attached to the armed conflict in Colombia and constitutes the focus of my work. Although this book is primarily concerned with cutaneous leishmaniasis, I will occasionally talk about mucosal leishmaniasis. While the mucosal form accounts for only 1–4 percent of all leishmaniasis cases in Colombia (INS 2017), the potential risk it poses to cutaneous leishmaniasis patients has been important for the overall management of the disease in the country (Pinto-García 2022).

Depending on the region, cutaneous leishmaniasis is popularly known in Colombia as *guaral*, *bejuco*, *yateví*, or *pito*. The most commonly used term is *pito*, especially in Caquetá, Putumayo, Guaviare, and Meta, which are zones where the armed conflict and the presence of guerrilla groups have been particularly prominent. The biomedical terminology used for the disease and the broad heterogeneity of nonbiomedical names reflect diverse experiences rather than a unified or uniform understanding (Pinto-García 2024).

The World Health Organization (WHO) considers leishmaniasis a "neglected tropical disease." Categorized as *tropical* and *neglected* and seen as a vector-borne skin disease exclusively affecting poor people in developing countries, leishmaniasis carries the labels through which tropical medicine, international health, and global health have become both famous and infamous in the context of imperialism and (neo)colonial expansion (Haraoui 2007; Benchimol and Jogas Junior 2020). Thus, this study of leishmaniasis and its war entanglements in Colombia dialogues with a growing list of works dealing with the past and current entanglements of colonialism, scientific research, and international (or global) health.[5] In the same vein, more recently, leishmaniasis has also been categorized as an *emerging disease*, which highlights its threatening potential to become an epidemic of global proportions. In biomedical accounts, tourism, military operations, and immigration from developing and leishmaniasis-endemic countries to developed and nonendemic ones have been described as a growing risk.[6] Thus, works that critically analyze the discourse of emerging diseases, its political and economic underpinnings, and its institutional deployments in the context of global health are also relevant to this project (French and Mykhalovskiy 2013; Lakoff 2010; King 2004, 2002). Although it is beyond the scope of this book, the emerging diseases discourse frames many of the connections among the local governance of leishmaniasis in Colombia, biomedical research on leishmaniasis conducted in the country, bilateral exchanges between the United States and Colombia, and the multilateral agenda of global health.

This has much to do with the fact that among infectious diseases, leishmaniasis—both cutaneous and visceral—stands out as a notorious public health problem in contexts recently affected by war and political terror, including the most recent episode of armed conflict in the Gaza Strip (Berry and Berrang-Ford 2016; Ghert-Zand 2024). For example, epidemiologists have attributed a major epidemic of visceral leishmaniasis in Sudan to the civil war that took place between 1983 and 2005 (J. Seaman, Mercer, and Sondorp 1996). In Iraq, war and instability are believed to be responsible for the increase in the number of visceral leishmaniasis cases (Jacobson 2011; Majeed et al. 2013). The largest outbreaks of cutaneous leishmaniasis in Afghanistan have taken place in Kabul refugee camps between 2002 and 2007, and the persistence of the disease has been attributed to the constant migration of people as a result of war (Aagaard-Hansen, Nombela, and Alvar 2010). While several outbreaks of leishmaniasis have occurred in the Middle East, mainly linked to war-associated population migration, the frequency and magnitude of outbreaks in the region have markedly increased with the Syrian war (Alawieh et al. 2014; Inci et al. 2015; Sharara and Kanj 2014). Several articles also report the drastic rise of leishmaniasis cases among foreign troops operating in the Middle East, especially members of the US Army participating in the so-called War on Terror (Beiter et al. 2019; Kitchen, Lawrence, and Coleman 2009; Lesho et al. 2004). In fact, by 2005, cutaneous leishmaniasis had become "the commonest global war on terror-associated reason for outpatient consultation" at the Walter Reed Army Medical Center in Bethesda, Maryland, US (Zapor and Moran 2005, 395; see also Profounda, Inc. 2023).

As such, the relationship between war and leishmaniasis in Colombia cannot be disassociated from broader connections between these two phenomena in other places. While the mechanisms and actors involved in the entanglements of war and leishmaniasis in other contexts differ significantly from the particularities I have traced in Colombia, connections can be established among localities, especially in light of global health regulations and the discourses that shape them. As the first in-depth ethnographic study of leishmaniasis and the first work in the social sciences investigating the relationship between this disease and the Colombian armed conflict, this book hopes to provoke further reflections and motivate additional and necessary research on the current links between infectious diseases and war in Colombia and beyond.

Pharmaceutical Treatment of Leishmaniasis

Leishmaniasis is labeled as a "neglected tropical disease" because it affects marginalized populations in developing contexts that do not represent a profitable market for pharmaceutical companies. As it entails a highly uncertain, risky, and time-consuming process that will not necessarily result in enough or immediate returns, the development of pharmaceuticals for diseases such as leishmaniasis tends to be regarded as an uninteresting business. This "innovation crisis" implies that the currently available antileishmanial drugs are not that different from the colonial pharmacopeia, including a collection of highly toxic, expensive, and obsolete drugs, most of which were developed to fight diseases other than leishmaniasis (Barbeitas 2019, 131).

Glucantime is the brand name of the standard drug used to treat leishmaniasis in Colombia and most Latin American countries. This highly toxic pharmaceutical is produced by the French multinational pharmaceutical company Sanofi. The standard treatment is systemic, which means that the drug is injected intramuscularly or intravenously and travels through the bloodstream, reaching all the cells of, and thus affecting, the entire body. While health care workers in countries such as Brazil have a marked preference for the intravenous administration of Glucantime, the standard practice in Colombia is to deliver this medicine intramuscularly—injected into the buttocks. The therapy involves a once-a-day administration of two injections, one in each buttock, over the course of twenty days (twenty-eight days in the case of mucosal leishmaniasis). The dose of Glucantime to be administered depends on the weight of the patient, with three to four ampoules per day being the usual dosage for adults.

Antimony is the active pharmaceutical ingredient in Glucantime. Most of the antimony in the world (84 percent) comes from 114 mines located in China, where antimony pollution in soils, sediments, water, and plants in the proximity of mining and smelting areas constitutes a major threat to environmental and human health (He et al. 2012). Today, this chemical is mainly used as a flame retardant incorporated into textiles, papers, adhesives, tires, brake linings, and plastics (He et al. 2012). Although the current use of antimony in medicine is marginal compared to this industrial application, its therapeutic history is much longer. In seventeenth-century Europe, the ability of antimony to provoke sweating, vomiting, and purging was seen as a valuable alternative to bloodletting, capable of expelling unwanted humors from the body (McCallum 1999). At that point in history, however, the toxic nature of this substance was already the subject of intense dispute among medical practitioners—particularly between Galenists and iatrochemists—who heatedly debated whether antimony should be accepted as a medicine or rejected as a poison (Debus 2001). The latter view prevailed, which is why the use of antimony in medicine declined in the following centuries. However, in the twentieth century, antimonials (antimony compounds) began to be used for the treatment of two parasitic diseases: leishmaniasis and schistosomiasis (Greenwood 2008). While less toxic and antimony-free alternatives were developed for the latter in the 1970s, the only medical application of this chemical element that persists today is in the pharmaceutical treatment of leishmaniasis (Sundar and Chakravarty 2010).

The twentieth-century history of the use of antimonials against leishmaniasis originated in Brazil. In 1905, an antimony-containing substance known as tartar emetic was shown to act against parasites that caused sleeping sickness in Africa (Haldar, Sen, and Roy 2011, 2). From a biomedical point of view, leishmaniasis, sleeping sickness, and Chagas disease are all caused by flagellated parasites known as trypanosomatid protozoa. This relatedness led Brazilian physician Gaspar Vianna to think that tartar emetic could also be useful to deal with parasites causing leishmaniasis. In 1912, he reported that tartar emetic injections were successfully used for the treatment of leishmaniasis in his country (Vianna 1912). Since then, antimonials have been the first-choice therapy against this disease. While less toxic antimonial compounds were developed in the 1920s (Haldar, Sen, and Roy 2011), substantial improvements have not been achieved since then. Significantly, toxicity remains the main problem of leishmaniasis pharmaceutical treatment today, which highlights the need to use and develop therapeutic alternatives (DNDi 2023; Organización Panamericana de la Salud 2013, vii).

In most countries where leishmaniasis is endemic, the public health strategy to manage the disease is primarily a therapeutic, pharmaceutical intervention. There is no preventive or therapeutic vaccine against any form of leishmaniasis, and its development is unlikely to materialize in the near future (see Kamhawi 2017). Despite their toxicity and severe poisonous effects primarily on the heart, liver, kidneys, and pancreas, antimonials continue to be used as standard first-line therapy against leishmaniasis. Sanofi and GlaxoSmithKline produce these drugs, commercially known as Glucantime and Pentostam, respectively. Although they are considered to have similar therapeutic efficacy, the current worldwide distribution of these pharmaceuticals is not uniform but instead mirrors a global geopolitical division inherited from World War II. According to one of the scientists who participated in the development of Pentostam in the UK: "War broke out in 1939 and there was a race to replace the essential drugs no longer available from Germany," including an antimonial drug called Solustibosan for the treatment of leishmaniasis (Goodwin 1995, 340). This led to the development of Pentostam by the British, and Glucantime by the French (Rath et al. 2003, 551). At the Wellcome Chemical Research Laboratory in London, William Solomon was in charge of testing different compounds on hamsters to find a replacement for Solustibosan. This work concluded in 1946 with the registration of a very similar molecule under the name of Pentostam (Barbeitas 2020). In the same year, Durand and his colleagues (1946) reported, for the first time, the successful use of meglumine antimoniate (Glucantime) to treat six patients suffering from leishmaniasis in France. Another clinical study on Glucantime appeared in the French literature in 1947 (Davis Marsden 1985, 187), and further trials were conducted in Italy in 1948, leading to the commercialization of the drug by a French company called Specia (Greenwood 2008, 309). Specia—Societé Parisienne d'Expansion Chimique—was a subsidiary of Poulenc Frères-Usine du Rhône, which later merged with an American and a German company to constitute the group Aventis in 1999. In 2004, Aventis merged with Sanofi, and Sanofi-Aventis emerged as one of the largest pharmaceutical companies in the world (Ravina 2011, 54). In 2011, Sanofi-Aventis changed its name to Sanofi.

Traditionally, countries that were under British influence have used Pentostam, and countries influenced by the French have preferred Glucantime (Barbeitas 2020, 19). In a similar vein, French- and Spanish-speaking countries like Colombia have conventionally used Glucantime, while Anglophone countries have traditionally chosen Pentostam (Wortmann et al. 2002, 261). In Brazil, the preference of Glucantime over Pentostam was also the result of the establishment in 1919 of a branch of the Poulenc company—Sanofi's predecessor—close to São Paulo. This probably helped facilitate the export of Glucantime to other Latin American countries and to standardize the use of this drug to treat leishmaniasis in places like Colombia (Barbeitas 2020, 19–20).

Besides antimonials, there are other pharmaceuticals currently available for the systemic treatment of leishmaniasis: an oral drug called miltefosine and two additional drugs called pentamidine and amphotericin B (conventional and liposomal). However, each of these medications has its drawbacks, which are mostly related to high levels of toxicity, long duration of the treatment, and high prices. In the case of pentamidine, Guillaume Lachenal (2017) reconstructed the downfall of this drug after it caused disastrous therapeutic "accidents" and many deaths in Africa, where it was used in the 1950s to prevent sleeping sickness. Thus, antimony-free antileishmanial drugs are not necessarily better than either Glucantime or Pentostam (Didwania et al. 2017). In fact, one of the statements I heard again and again at the 2017 World-Leish conference was that there is to date no satisfactory drug for leishmaniasis and the current set of options to treat the disease will remain the same for quite some time.

In Colombia, vector-control strategies are nearly absent from the state management of leishmaniasis made available to the general population. As such, the public health management of leishmaniasis in Colombia is almost exclusively centered on Glucantime. Primarily because of their high cost, the use of treatments other than Glucantime is the exception, not the rule. In practice, the use of these other drugs is considered only under specific patient conditions such as therapeutic failure; that is, the persistence of skin ulcers despite Glucantime treatment (MinSalud 2023, 12–13). As I show in the following pages, nonmilitary populations have historically faced multiple access barriers to Glucantime that the state had put in place during wartime and maintains to this day, even after reaching a peace agreement with the FARC. If this is the first-line therapy option, the use of more expensive and less available second-line therapies is even more marginal. This means that the people who manage to access medical care and treatment for leishmaniasis are generally treated with Glucantime and hardly ever with miltefosine, pentamidine, or amphotericin B.

In particular, the current guideline recommends the use of miltefosine as second-line therapy for adults and first-line therapy for children (MinSalud

2023, 12–13). Yet this drug is rarely prescribed in Colombia because it is usually unavailable and too costly for the state. According to Ministry of Health officials interviewed in 2017, miltefosine costs six times more than Glucantime. As the first oral medication for cutaneous leishmaniasis, many biomedical scientists are miltefosine enthusiasts. However, this pharmaceutical product remains a very toxic drug and is also a systemic treatment that affects the whole body. While the development of miltefosine for the treatment of leishmaniasis was the result of a 1995 public-private agreement between WHO and a pharmaceutical company called Asta Medica, the drug's ownership rights have been exchanged many times among four pharmaceutical companies through business mergers and acquisitions (Barbeitas 2020). Under the brand name Impavido, miltefosine was sold by Asta Medica to Zentaris, then resold by Zentaris to Paladin, then by Paladin to Knight Therapeutics. In the United States, it has been marketed by Profounda since 2016. As a result, miltefosine's "public vocation" has been almost completely lost. Its price is now very high, the current owner (Knight Therapeutics) is not keen on making it accessible, and many leishmaniasis-endemic countries—like Colombia—have not been able to sustain the availability of this drug (Barbeitas 2020; Pinto-García 2016).

The Colombian Army, which represents the population with the best access to antileishmanial drugs in Colombia, has always employed Glucantime as the first-line therapy for leishmaniasis. Within this institution, pentamidine is employed after a failed Glucantime treatment. As a "second-rate medicine, used mainly in the periphery of the Western World" (Lachenal 2017, 17), pentamidine is also a drug of dubious benefit. If this pharmaceutical does not work, soldiers are systemically treated with amphotericin B. Unfortunately, this medicine is also highly toxic and expensive.

The Pharmaceuticalization of War

The notion of social determinants has been important to label how the conflict has a bearing on leishmaniasis in Colombia—but no more than that. Under this paradigm, medical care and health technologies by themselves are considered insufficient to solve a public health problem. Instead, social factors take a far more important place in understanding the fundamental causes of disease and health disparities, as well as in thinking about possible solutions (Braveman and Gottlieb 2014). On the other hand, STS scholars have been more interested in studying how health technologies such as pharmaceuticals are multilayered objects whose success or failure (or something in between) depends on the social context in which they are embedded. In an effort to bring these literatures on social determinants and STS closer together, Stefan Timmermans and Rebecca Kaufman (2020) have highlighted the value of studying the effects of technologies on health disparities. They invite STS to pay more attention to the ways in which health technologies not only reconfigure health practices and subjectivities but also stratify societies. From this perspective, technologies are not assumed to be an essential part of the problem or the solution of inequality from the outset. On the contrary: they become an object of study.

Anthropologist João Biehl (2007) provides a remarkable example of such an approach. He studied the rollout of antiretroviral therapy (ART) in Brazil that was initiated in 1996, a state policy that was widely celebrated for demonstrating that extensive provision of drugs for HIV-positive people was possible in developing countries. While Biehl acknowledges that this strategy brought remarkable improvements in access to therapy for thousands of people and significantly reduced mortality rates, he warns that such a drug-centered public health model tends to marginalize preventive strategies. Moreover, it overlooks improvements in medical care, health infrastructure, and general well-being, which ultimately depend on alleviating poverty, balancing inequalities, and addressing human rights violations. This *pharmaceuticalization of public health*, he argues, is especially detrimental to the most vulnerable people living with HIV because the state's presence comes in the form of pharmaceuticals but not as a strengthened public health system capable of supporting the sustained provision of medications and other nonpharmaceutical aspects that are also crucial to leading healthy and dignified lives. This type of public health approach has been shown to be particularly prominent in Global South contexts, where health problems are often framed in terms of lack of pharmaceuticals, reducing the scope of public health strategies and the range of possible solutions to simply the provision of drugs (Pollock 2011; Ecks 2005).[7]

In Colombia, it is not an overstatement to say that the state management of leishmaniasis starts and ends with Glucantime. A *pharmaceuticalized* model of public health that relies almost exclusively on this drug displaces preventive strategies and ignores broader issues of economic inequality and marginalization that are central to the occurrence of the disease among those who inhabit poor and remote areas of the country (Pinto-García 2022). More perturbingly, this book shows that Glucantime is officially delivered through a complex control scheme that, relying on regulations, institutions, discourses, expertise, and knowledges, serves to manage populations and produce therapeutic distinctions between state allies (Army soldiers) and state enemies (guerrilla members and civilians with uncertain affiliations) in the context of the armed conflict.

Thus, my work illustrates that Glucantime is not an apolitical or neutral entity, nor is it a predetermined technology that solves a public health problem in foreseeable ways. In fact, this drug does much more—and much less—than simply fulfill its assigned therapeutic purpose. Together with rifles, land mines, military uniforms, and many other objects typically belonging to warfare, Glucantime is a pharmaceutical that has made the Colombian armed conflict "*materially* thick" (Widger 2018, 397). The state has weaponized Glucantime and remade it into a valuable biopolitical instrument of war by restricting its circulation and accessibility according to a social order of included allies and excluded foes that is rooted in the armed conflict. Crucially, the pharmaceuticalization of public health in the case of Colombian leishmaniasis operates as an underlying condition for such a process. In other words, the pharmaceuticalization of public health provides the context for the expansion of pharmaceutical technologies into war-making processes—what I call the *pharmaceuticalization of war.*

As a biopolitical instrument of war, Glucantime works beyond the realm and concerns of medical practice and authority, sustaining the internal enemy ideology and the social divisions established in wartime. Any person with leishmaniasis seeking medical care from the state gets channeled into the Glucantime regime and ends up encountering a war regime. On the one hand, those considered enemies (guerrillas) or potential enemies of the state (civilians with uncertain affiliations) are excluded from access to *the* pharmaceutical that encapsulates the state's response to leishmaniasis. On the other hand, those considered allies of the state (soldiers) are included and protected in the form of pharmaceutical care. Thus, a significant portion of the following pages is devoted to Glucantime and the various ways in which this pharmaceutical object is embroiled in the *maraña* formed by leishmaniasis and conflict through the pharmaceuticalization of war.

The notion of *pharmaceuticalization* is a further development of *medicalization*, an older but key concept in the sociology of health and illness that has theoretically underpinned important scholarship since the 1970s (Abraham 2010; S. E. Bell and Figert 2012). Medicalization has been primarily concerned with medicine as an institution of expanding social control that makes "the labels 'healthy' and 'ill' *relevant* to an ever increasing part of human existence" (Zola 1972, 487). The concept of medicalization has been helpful in thinking critically about instances in which a nonmedical problem is defined in medical terms or when medical interventions are presented as solutions (Conrad 2005). Relatedly, *pharmaceuticalization* denotes the increasingly frequent tendency of using pharmaceuticals to address a broad variety of problems and situations, even nonmedical ones (Williams, Martin, and Gabe 2011). Studies that trace pharmaceuticalization think of the growing role of pharmaceuticals in society as "a dynamic and complex heterogeneous socio-technical process" that involves the expansion of *pharmaceutical regimes* (Williams, Martin, and Gabe 2011, 721). "That is to say that it can be understood as a network of institutions, organisations, actors, and artefacts, alongside those cognitive structures and affective processes associated with the creation, production and use of therapeutics" (Gabe et al. 2015, 193). Thus, scholarly projects interested in pharmaceuticalization processes pay attention to the participation of a heterogeneous array of entities, practices, knowledges, and emotions in the colonization of everyday life by pharmaceuticals.

The leading influence of pharmaceutical companies on the growing presence of pharmaceutical products in society has been the focus of most studies on pharmaceuticalization (for instance, Dumit 2012). Thus, the concept has been primarily employed to make sense of cases where pharmaceutical companies, seeking to expand their market, develop or repurpose drugs for conditions that were previously unrecognized as pathological or in need of a pharmaceutical fix. In that vein, pharmaceuticalization has been particularly fruitful in studying the use of drugs as psychosocial remedies for sexual problems, sleep disorders, hyperactivity, anxiety, attention deficits, and depression (Abraham 2010). However, other scholars have documented pharmaceuticalization processes developing in arenas where the pharmaceutical industry does not necessarily play a dominant role. Understood as "the translation or transformation of human conditions, capabilities and capacities into opportunities for pharmaceutical intervention" (Williams, Martin, and Gabe 2011, 711), pharmaceuticalization has been increasingly useful to make sense of phenomena taking place far beyond the medical profession and the pharmaceutical industry (McReynolds-Perez 2014). Elbe and colleagues (2015), for example, have drawn attention to the role that governments play in creating regulatory conditions and policy instruments for the expansion of pharmaceuticals in society. Fearing the possibility of pandemics and bioterrorist attacks, these authors show how, under a health security discourse, governments in the United States and Europe have acquired and stockpiled enormous amounts of pharmaceuticals, as well as promoted the development of new medical countermeasures. They argue that "governments too are today accelerating, intensifying and opening up new trajectories of pharmaceuticalization in society" (Elbe, Roemer-Mahler, and Long 2015, 263). Similarly, this book documents a case in which the role of the pharmaceutical industry or the medical establishment in the pharmaceuticalization process is not as relevant as the practices, visions, and logic of a state at war.

In Colombia, the restricted paths through which Glucantime circulates naturalize leishmaniasis as a guerrilla disease, differentiate the population along friend/foe lines, and stabilize social orders and forms of control engendered by the war. Paraphrasing Didier Fassin (2008, 160), Glucantime *catalyzes*—in the sense that this drug not only unveils historical tensions in conflict-ridden Colombia but also contributes to producing them by forcing people to one side or the other of the state war against guerrillas. This pattern of inclusion/exclusion that plays into the access to leishmaniasis treatments is a telling sign that the ordering of societies at war can also be found in conventionally and nominally peaceful domains such as science, technology, and public health. This coevolution of a pharmaceutical regime and wartime social orders is what I call the *pharmaceuticalization of war*. This notion foregrounds the processes through which wartime social orders and pharmaceutical regimes are mutually constituted. Under these premises, this book tells a story about both the penetration of pharmaceutical products into war-making processes and the fashioning of the war apparatus to fit the constraints of a therapeutic regime primarily based on Glucantime. While this is not totally unlike the simultaneous *militarization of medicine* and *medicalization of war* suggested by Mark Harrison (1996), the *pharmaceuticalization of war* lays primary emphasis on the crucial participation of pharmaceuticals in armed conflicts and the coconstitution of wartime social orders and pharmaceutical regimes.

There are two main types of violence produced by the pharmaceuticalization of war. While it generates exclusion from access to the drug that the state uses to address leishmaniasis, the high toxicity of Glucantime also affects the health of the few who do have access to it. As chapter 4 shows, this is especially true for soldiers of the Colombian Army, who may receive up to six treatments for leishmaniasis during their years in the military. To put this another way, the pharmaceuticalization of war produces violence by default and by excess of medication. As such, the toxicity associated with the use of antileishmanial pharmaceuticals amid armed conflict is also a significant component of the *maraña*.

Embedded in a world that is permanently contaminated, STS scholars have paid close attention to the inescapable nature of toxic exposures that characterizes our present. The ubiquity of these chemicals makes the resulting human and animal health problems so diverse, multiple, and interrelated that it is virtually impossible to pinpoint the precise causes, magnitudes, and temporalities of the problem and, thus, to identify culprits and demand redress (Nading 2020). But the damage caused by toxic exposures is not evenly distributed, as Liboiron, Tironi, and Calvillo (2018) argue. While we all share a condition in which life is permanently altered by chemical exposures, toxicity does not affect us all equally because it is "located in specific territories and premised upon and reproduced by systems of colonialism, racism, capitalism, patriarchy, and other structures that require land and bodies as sacrifice zones" (Liboiron, Tironi, and Calvillo 2018, 332). As such, toxic harm is best understood as a system that alters order and relationships at one level but maintains structures of inequality and sacrifice at another, which is a defining aspect of many forms of violence, including war (Liboiron, Tironi, and Calvillo 2018).

While pharmaceuticals usually enter our bodies with greater consent than environmental pollutants, the toxicity they carry is also distributed unevenly, reproducing inequalities and structures of power (Langston 2010). In conflict-torn Colombia, the bodies most affected by the Glucantime-based system of toxic harm are those of young men from poor, often rural and racialized backgrounds who join the military out of obligation or necessity. Their antileishmanial treatment has a coercive character since refusal to receive it would mean dismissal from the institution. The lower ranks of the Army are populated by bodies considered both essential and disposable. The pharmacological wear and tear that the state and society impose on these bodies is not included in the accounting of war. Soldiers' heart arrhythmias, their weakened pancreas, their inability to reproduce, and the pounds of weight they will never regain are not counted in the cost of war. Nor are they found in the public condemnation of violence or in the scientific articles published by Colombian researchers. Cynthia Enloe writes that "war-waging governments depend on us to *not* count the wounded" (2023, 84). The Colombian state also relies on us not paying attention to the soldiers who have become pharmacological casualties in the name of leishmaniasis, a disease they acquire while making war happen.

War and Disease

"*Somos una sociedad enferma*" (We are a sick society). This statement is commonly heard in Colombia in reference to everyday crimes, human rights violations, and expressions of war that Colombians have seen populating the news day by day, for many decades. The sickness refers to the naturalization of violence, a deep damage—a kind of profound and unspeakable inadequacy that translates into a shortage of empathy and compassion. I am not saying that we Colombians are naturally, essentially, or inevitably violent or indolent. But our society has been profoundly transformed and fragmented by the armed conflict, so much that it is still very hard for us, even today, to understand and agree on the magnitude of what has happened, how we all have directly or indirectly participated, and what is needed to put a final stop to violence, heal the wounds, and avoid repetitions.

Arguably, we still do not fully grasp how war has made us sick, how we have become sick *from* war. Although the armed conflict is Colombia's most prominent problem and probably the most-researched subject in the country (Blair Trujillo 2009; F. E. González 2003), there is very little work developed about the links between health and the war. The Truth Commission (Comisión para el Esclarecimiento de la Verdad, la Convivencia y la No Repetición, hereafter CEV) established in 2017 made an unprecedented effort to document and make visible aspects of that relationship along three main lines: acts of violence against health personnel, the use of health care infrastructures to wage war, and the diversion of public health care funds for warfare and illegal purposes (CEV 2021). Yet our understanding of how violence has been nurturing and producing disease over many years of war is still egregiously incomplete.[8]

While this book is very much concerned with bodily marks left by war, structural violence, and the implications of armed conflict on health institutions, access, and workers, it takes a different approach. It focuses on a single disease—cutaneous leishmaniasis. Of course, this is not the only illness affecting members of the different armies who have historically confronted each other in Colombia, from soldiers of the state military forces to far-right paramilitaries to far-left guerrillas. For example, malaria, gastrointestinal infections, and urinary infections (in the case of female guerrillas) have also been very common (Orjuela Benavides 2017). However, I have decided to pay close attention to this noncontagious, nondeadly, and curable skin disease because it is highly emblematic and illustrative of the complicated *enmarañamiento* among biomedicine, public health, and war in the Colombian context. The very nature and epidemiology of leishmaniasis is rather unremarkable and encourages forgetfulness—as was the case with the Spanish flu pandemic during the First World War until the recent emergence of COVID-19 (Crosby 2003). And yet I show how an infectious disease that may not be so extraordinary or deserving of public and international attention can be so revealing about the entanglements of warfare and medicine in contemporary times.

As it is well acknowledged, diseases, not battlefield injuries, have been the primary cause of casualties and deaths in many armed conflict contexts throughout history. This is especially true for infectious diseases whereby pathogens—parasites, bacteria, or viruses—have affected and decimated populations of civilians and combatants in past and present contexts of war.[9] Among infectious diseases, those transmitted by insects have often been shown to be determinant for the course and outcome of wars at different points in time.[10] By recognizing war as a highly disruptive process that impacts health in very diverse and contextual ways, critical medical anthropologists have ethnographically explored illness, public health, and clinical practice in contexts of conflict. They have examined the specific mechanisms through which war and disease have become inextricably entangled in certain settings, unveiling costs of war that, in more widespread narratives around conflict, tend to remain hidden.[11] Although I draw inspiration from these works, this book takes into deep consideration the knowledge-making practices and institutions as well as the technologies, infrastructures, and regulations that mediate the experience of a disease unfolding in the midst of armed conflict.

In war contexts, ill health is often worsened by food and pharmaceutical blockades, disruption of public health programs, militarized health care, attacks on health personnel, and intentional destruction of health care infrastructures. The current wars in Sudan and Ukraine, for example, confirm that armed conflicts almost invariably go hand in hand with epidemic outbreaks and health crises that severely compound rampant violence (Ogao 2023; Kellman 2022; Kluger and Law 2022). Although today's world is increasingly marked by armed conflicts and epidemics, the intersection of warfare and infectious diseases is a crucial field of inquiry that has not received enough attention from STS ethnographers.[12] This has become all the more urgent and notorious in view of the multiple forms of militarization associated with state control of the COVID-19 pandemic (Diaz and Mountz 2020), mainly in contexts historically marked by conflict and a tremendous amount of power and resources concentrated in military and police forces (Ojeda and Pinto-García 2020; M. Parker, MacGregor, and Akello 2020).

My analysis develops in close dialogue with ethnographies that have interrogated the links among war, embodiment, biomedicine, and public health. Although the works of Kenneth T. MacLeish (2013) and Zoë Wool (2015) are not entirely concerned with health, their ethnographic explorations of the ordinary life of American soldiers and veterans constitute remarkable examples of scholarship that, partially drawing on STS theoretical contributions, study the bodily dimensions and everyday realities of those whose job it is to make war happen. Wool explores what it means to lead an ordinary life in the aftermath of war, amid the precariousness and physical and mental damage produced by extraordinary forms of violence. MacLeish's ethnography is particularly useful for making sense of the biopolitical condition of soldiers, a group of people rendered vulnerable for "living in and with bodies that are instruments and objects of violence" (2013, 13). Through careful documentation of the war-making experiences of active members of the US Army, MacLeish shows that war is a never-ending phenomenon that permeates various aspects of society. Both Wool and MacLeish make clear that it is impossible to draw a line between the state armed forces and the rest of society or to demarcate the spatial, temporal, cultural, and bodily boundaries where war begins and where it ends. This book is also attentive to the experiences of those whose bodies are harmed while making war happen as well as civilians immersed in spaces, rationales, and practices shaped by the war. I show that leishmaniasis is not only one of the ordinary ways in which the war affects and alters the lives of combatants and civilians in Colombian war zones; it is also an embodied condition that moves the conflict to places where its presence is unexpected. Bodies affected by both leishmaniasis and the war also inhabit the domains of public health, medicine, and biomedical research, where epistemic and technological dimensions become much more conspicuous than in either MacLeish's or Wool's publications.

In that sense, this book is also in dialogue with the work of Jennifer Terry (2017), who has turned her analytical attention to the intersection between biomedicine and war in the post-9/11 context of US-led combat operations in Iraq and Afghanistan. She is especially interested in the development of new biomedical technologies in the US and how these are enmeshed in warfare discourses and practices, acting within but also far beyond the contours of military institutions. The term *bioinequality* holds an important place in Terry's account, as it highlights that "bodies suffering from war wounds are classified by a variety of social technologies" that value some lives over others (2017, 20). As a result, the benefits and promises of new therapies, devices, and pharmaceuticals developed thanks to—and in the name of—war are available to some but are denied to most people.

While Terry is mostly concerned with "the biomedical industry's development of high-tech, expensive, and lifelong therapies that are too costly for the vast majority of persons wounded in war" (2017, 21), my case shows that even old, state-provided, and highly deficient technologies—like Glucantime—can be used to redraw distinctions between people in societies at war. The instrumentalization of pharmaceuticals that I document in this book resonates with Joseph Masco's work (2014), in which he argues that weapons are not the only means of violence that the state monopolizes. Affects, imaginaries, infrastructures, and other elements of the material world are also part of the state's arsenal to produce violence. This book makes evident how the state control of a pharmaceutical to generate distinctions between state allies and enemies in a context of war exemplifies the ways in which medications can also participate in the perpetration of state violence.

The instrumentalization of drugs in war contexts is not necessarily new or unique to Colombia. In his study of the rise and fall of state medicine in Iraq, Omar Dewachi has documented that, in the aftermath of the 1991 Gulf War, this country was subjected to a series of international sanctions that prohibited, among others, the import of crucial antibiotics "due to their 'dual use' for military and civilian purposes" (Dewachi 2017, xi). The UN claimed that the goal was to destroy Iraq's military capacity after its occupation of Kuwait in 1990 by "severing the 'supply lines' on which the Iraqi regime depended" (Dewachi 2017, 7). Dewachi has characterized these restrictions on access to medications and other goods needed for the reconstruction of Iraq as "one of the harshest experiments of the war under UN economic sanctions" (2017, ix). The implication of pharmaceuticals in warfare that I explore in this book is yet another example of the dramatic consequences that such a vicious strategy can have—not only for combatants but also for civilians.

The Colombian Armed Conflict

For more than six decades, Colombia has experienced a tragic war. The Colombian armed conflict is a very complex and prolonged phenomenon that has caused 269,285 deaths between 1958 and June 30, 2023 (Observatorio de Memoria y Conflicto 2023). Civilians account for 81.5 percent of these deaths, and the war has caused more than 9.5 million victimizing events, both fatal and nonfatal.[13] Its beginning dates back to 1946 when a wave of violence started between the two major traditional parties—liberal and conservative. What began as a bipartisan political struggle took on new political nuances as the international setting shifted after World War II. The consolidation of socialism in the Soviet Union, the ideological and geopolitical divisions during the Cold War, the imperialist strategies of the United States, and the triumph of the Cuban Revolution in 1959 acquired significant relevance in many Latin American countries. In the 1960s, after an agreement between liberal and conservative representatives to alternate power every four years during the period between 1958 and 1974, several leftist guerrilla groups emerged in Colombia to rebel against the ruling elites and the country's profound inequalities, especially those related to land distribution. While some of these groups signed peace agreements with the government in the early 1990s, and one of them—the Movimiento 19 de Abril, or M-19—even had a leading role in the enactment of the constitution that has governed the Colombian nation since 1991, others continued fighting against the military forces of the state.

In the 1980s, the illegal drug business took off and, merging into an already heated environment, provided favorable conditions and the economic means for the escalation of armed confrontations. The illicit economy of cocaine allowed for the strengthening of the FARC and the National Liberation Army (Ejército de Liberación Nacional, or ELN). These guerrilla groups also started using extortive kidnapping of wealthy people—including drug lords—as a means of financial support. Drug cartels, leftist guerrillas, economic interests, and regional political elites became entwined in a seemingly endless swirl of violence and corruption. The parallel consolidation of right-wing paramilitary groups during these years took on unprecedented proportions in 1997 with their unification under the name United Self-Defenders of Colombia (Autodefensas Unidas de Colombia, or AUC). The AUC were established as an armed force to fight guerrillas and end any expression of leftist ideology in Colombia. They were sponsored by corporations, ranchers, large landowners, and drug traffickers and often operated in collusion with the state and its armed forces. While guerrilla organizations had an antistate character and sought to destroy the state to create something new, the paramilitaries' aim was to maintain the status quo and co-opt the state (Avila 2019, 34–35).

Since the 1980s, the escalation of the Colombian armed conflict has been remarkable, especially under the government formed by Álvaro Uribe, who was elected president for two terms (2002–2006 and 2006–2010). He galvanized the idea that the military solution—more war against the war—was the only possible path toward the end of armed violence. A pivotal moment in the war trajectory came when Uribe launched an unprecedented military offensive against guerrilla groups—primarily against the FARC—through a policy called Defense and Democratic Security (Política de Defensa y Seguridad Democrática, or PSD). In the context of the long-standing war on drugs and the burgeoning war on terror, antiterrorist discourses in relation to guerrilla groups were greatly emphasized during Uribe's government to obtain international support to wipe out both insurgencies and cocaine production. Borrowing terminology from the US Drug Enforcement Administration (DEA), Uribe no longer spoke of guerrillas but of "narcoterrorists" (Andreas 2020). Under Uribe's government, the number of soldiers in the Army increased by 31.6 percent (Leal Buitrago 2011). Between 2003 and 2009, the state went from spending nine to almost twenty trillion pesos in security and defense (Angarita 2011, 294). Also, new mobile brigades were created, joint forces commands were implemented, and military operations were technologically strengthened. Consequently, the Army ceased to be reactive and began to take the initiative in operational terms (E. Cruz 2015).

Although guerrillas have traditionally occupied many kinds of rural areas—particularly the jungle—under Uribe's government, the Army and paramilitary groups forced them to retreat and concentrate in the nation's forested environments. Guerrillas also modified their strategy by prioritizing intermittent sabotages and ambushes—actions more typical of guerrilla warfare, reminiscent of the guerrillas' military strategies in the initial stages of the armed conflict. The guerrilla modus operandi became all about causing exasperation and wearing out the opponent physically and emotionally to maximize casualties and strategic gains at the lowest possible operational cost. Additionally, given its military inferiority, guerrillas opted to limit their territorial control over strategic corridors, mainly with the extensive use of land mines and similar explosive devices (CNMH and Fundación Prolongar 2017; Echandía Castilla and Bechara Gómez 2006).

Two elements of Uribe's military strategy are particularly important to understanding the *maraña* formed by leishmaniasis and war in Colombia. First, with the growth of the Army and the development of massive and several-month incursions into the jungles, the disease began to critically affect the Army in terms of the military capacity to fight the war (chapter 3). As I highlight throughout this book, this had a large impact on how leishmaniasis was managed within and beyond the Army. Second, Uribe used a warmongering and incendiary discourse against the guerrillas and also—and with devastating consequences—against social movements; groups defending social and environmental justice; human rights defenders; and, in general, any critic of his government and the power structures in Colombia. Dangerously, guerrillas, labeled as terrorists, were conflated with any person, group, or expression that was not aligned with the status quo or Uribe's actions and goals (E. Cruz 2015; Gallón 2005). This type of stigmatization was not new in Colombia and had a longer trajectory rooted in the National Security Doctrine expanded by the United States throughout Latin America during the Cold War. However, Uribe's PSD has been seen as an actualization of this doctrine and a continuation of the anticommunist bias beyond the Cold War era (Angarita 2011). "In fact, the PSD was aimed at the integration of society with an anti-terrorist purpose, calling into question the distinction between combatants and non-combatants" (Cruz 2016, 78).

Part of my argument is that the understanding of leishmaniasis as a typical guerrilla disease, combined with the visible lesions left by this disease on the skin, merged in such a way that these bodily marks have worked as actual stigmas singling out "enemies" of the state, those barely discernible from regular citizens. In the Colombian armed conflict, where distinctions between combatants and civilians have become so blurry, especially under Uribe's administration, guerrillas have been equated to terrorists, and any anti-establishment manifestation has been equated to terrorism or guerrilla warfare. As leishmaniasis sufferers have also been equated to guerrilla members, they have similarly become targets of state and paramilitary violence. Thus, in a country where guerrillas have been throughout decades consistently demonized as the primary enemy of the state, carrying a leishmaniasis sore can become life-threatening, as I explore in chapter 1.

Since 1982, there have been several attempts to reach a negotiated peace agreement between the state and the FARC guerrilla organization. In 2012, peace dialogues between the FARC and the government of Juan Manuel Santos were launched in Havana, Cuba. After almost four years of negotiations, FARC leader Rodrigo Londoño (better known by his war name 'Timochenko') and President Santos signed the peace accords in Cartagena, Colombia, on September 26, 2016. Less than a week later, the plebiscite seeking popular support for the ratification of the final agreement was rejected, with 50.2 percent of the population voting against it. This situation left the country in a political limbo from which the incumbent government came out weakened, and the right-wing opposition—led by then-senator and former president Álvaro Uribe—strengthened. The government devised a quick solution to this unsettling situation by signing a revised version of the peace deal on November 24, 2016, which was ratified by Congress less than a week later. Finally, there was a peace agreement in place, but the popular and political support across society was—and still is—far from uniform. During the negotiations, peace became a highly contentious issue, and, with the plebiscite results, the subsequent implementation of the peace agreements suffered even more from this polarization within Colombian society. There has not been enough political will or funds to carry out a process of the necessary dimensions, a situation that was already apparent under the administration that signed the peace agreement—the political context in which I developed my fieldwork.

The chances for a successful peace-building process were further diminished when Iván Duque, the presidential candidate supported by the group opposing the agreement, came to power in the years 2018–2022. The Kroc Institute for International Peace Studies, based at the University of Notre Dame in the United States, was appointed by the Colombian government and the FARC to verify and monitor the progress of the fifteen-year implementation of the peace agreement. Its latest and most recent report, published in June 2023, shows that only 20 percent of the commitments are at an intermediate level of implementation, while 37 percent and 13 percent of them are in a state of minimal or uninitiated implementation, respectively. While the peace agreement implementation showed a linear upward trend since its signing, the pace of implementation slowed down significantly in 2019 (Kroc Institute 2023, 3). Despite the fact that former FARC fighters formed a political party with seats in Congress and that the homicide rate in 2017 was the lowest in forty-two years (*El Espectador* 2018), the Colombian people are still struggling to build peace amid continuing violence, the rearmament of some FARC ex-combatants, and insufficient efforts to materialize the agreements.

Compared to the negotiation period that preceded the signing of the peace deal, violence has escalated in recent years. Despite the inauguration in August 2022 of the first leftist government in Colombian history, led by Gustavo Petro, this reality has not radically changed.

Between October 2016 and December 2017, amid this uncertain transition period from war to peace, I embarked on a path to explore the connections among health regulations, health care practices, war strategies, and violence-shaped science and technology. I could not have performed the field research to investigate the relationship between leishmaniasis and the Colombian war without the guarantees of the peace agreement. Practicing ethnography in such a context—negotiating access to a variety of field sites, traveling through conflict-ridden territories, conducting participant observation and in-depth interviews with victims and actors from different sides of the conflict—shaped the modes of inquiry I adopted, the conversations I engaged with, and the broad spectrum of emotions I experienced as an ethnographer in her homeland. In other words, this ethnography is both a product uniquely enabled by the transition as well as a reflection of the struggles that characterize it. Although I was able to do ethnographic research because of the promises, imaginaries, and materialities of peace, I also struggled to see peace, avoid violence, and open up spaces of hope for myself and others.

Tracing the *Maraña*

I became interested in leishmaniasis and its *enmarañamiento* with war when, in 2012, I was working on the administrative team of a Colombian research institution dedicated primarily to the biomedical study of this disease. After some months of working there, I was astounded to overhear—in a casual hallway conversation, no less—that Glucantime was restrictively controlled by the state as a means to harm guerrillas. To my surprise, I was also told that many of the patients who approached the institute's clinical facilities were commonly involved in activities considered to be illegal—often guerrilla members or coca harvesters, known locally as *raspachines*. I became especially intrigued by the way in which the restriction of Glucantime was assumed by scientists as something wrong but somehow conceivable, imaginable, and *normal* in the context of everyday violence in Colombia.

Through preliminary research, I understood that the relationship between leishmaniasis and the armed conflict had remained for the most part unwritten and undocumented. This also made me aware of the necessity of adopting ethnographic methodologies to document the more surreptitious narratives, experiences, and practices associated with the disease and the Colombian war.

Journalists have sporadically raised concerns about leishmaniasis and its connections to the armed conflict. Yet there has been no systematic effort to unravel the multiple relationships between the disease and the conflict, and neither scholars nor journalists have offered an in-depth analysis that is informed by the everyday experience, history, politics, and social dynamics of war.

Because Glucantime is not easily accessible, there is a question about whether or not it has been instrumentalized for war purposes.[14] The question, however, is sometimes simplistically explained away as a myth—something that people believe in but that does not reflect the free and timely distribution of the drug by the Ministry of Health and its subordinate institutions.[15] Since it is a thorny issue that might be interpreted as a war crime under international humanitarian law, both journalists and scientists are rather reluctant to point fingers or make accusations when the issue is brought up. Despite being a *secreto a voces*—a well-known secret, what Taussig (1999) would refer to as a "public secret"—the "facts" underlying the Glucantime restrictive control and its warfare uses cannot be found in a state policy or public documents and will hardly be verbalized as such by any public health officer or Army commander. This does not mean, however, that such a reality does not exist or that it is untraceable.

A major challenge is that it is difficult to encounter a leishmaniasis case in any clinic or health center, even in those medical facilities located close to endemic areas. In addition, leishmaniasis remains a marginal disease in medical practice and training, even in places like Colombia, which also limits the circulation of discourses about this illness. As a result, I have pieced together a picture of Colombian leishmaniasis from data I have gathered in sites where leishmaniasis cases and narratives ordinarily concentrate. In Colombia, biomedical research and the armed conflict serve as two distinct "magnets" attracting, concentrating, and articulating leishmaniasis experiences and discourses. I draw on these two magnetic poles to trace a path of ethnographic inquiry, constructing the multisited space of my research by following the disease through locations where it is traceable in everyday existence (Marcus 1995; Fortun 2009).

While treading on the heels of the disease, I quickly noticed that it was impossible to observe and discuss the experience of leishmaniasis sufferers without observing and discussing their therapeutic itineraries and their (mis)encounters with antileishmanial treatments, particularly Glucantime. To put it otherwise, I was confirming the persistent interdependence of the natural, the social, and the material (Latour 1992). Understanding the fluid presence and absence of this drug became a constant element of my ethnographic trajectory. Thus, while I followed leishmaniasis, I also ended up taking a biographical approach to Glucantime, tracing the various paths through which this pharmaceutical circulates across different contexts, staging a diverse cast of actors, and enacting various regimes of values (Van der Geest, Whyte, and Hardon 1996). Recognizing medications as products and producers of human culture, I have employed Glucantime as a useful sampling device for understanding the critical involvement of medications in the reciprocal production of war and leishmaniasis in Colombia (Charles Rosenberg, cited by Greene and Sismondo 2015, 5).

My ethnographic fieldwork began two weeks after FARC leader 'Timochenko' and President Santos signed the peace accords. Carolyn Nordstrom (2004) writes that we lack a proper term to describe the political reality that follows the end of an armed conflict. "Not-war-not-peace" seems to be a suitable name to portray this state of affairs. "Essentially it is a time when military actions occur that in and of themselves would be called 'war' or 'low-intensity-warfare,' but are not so labeled because they are hidden by a peace process no one wants to admit is failing" (Nordstrom 2004, 166–67). I conducted fourteen months of field research between October 2016 and December 2017, in the early stages of the not-war-not-peace period that continues to unfold as I write this book. I had developed a project to study the entanglements of leishmaniasis and war, but I soon realized that my research would turn out to be about an illness across an unfinished conflict and a nascent, partial, and still very precarious peace. Thus my fieldwork turned into a daily and embodied corroboration that "peace is never clearly distinct from war" and "is not a separate end point to achieve in time or space" (Koopman 2017, 1). At each of my field sites, I experienced this ambiguous reality, a mixture of sober optimism and nonnaive pessimism that my research participants—most of whom had been living in proximity to war—kept nurturing with their skeptical narratives, at times sweetened by sparks of hope.

I spent three months doing fieldwork at the Army's Leishmaniasis Recovery Center (Centro de Recuperación de la Leishmaniasis, hereafter CRL), sometimes called the Leishmaniasis Rehabilitation Center. This one-of-a-kind clinical facility, located within the Silva Plazas Battalion on the outskirts of Duitama, Boyacá, was established in the mid-2000s for the exclusive treatment and recovery of soldiers affected by the disease (fig. I.2). Right before I started my fieldwork at the CRL, in October 2016, all Glucantime treatments conducted by the Army were centralized at this clinical facility, which implied that during my time there, the vast majority of leishmaniasis cases in the Army were medically handled in this facility. Before that, Glucantime was also administered at the Tolemaida Military Regional Hospital (Tolima) and the Military District in Carepa (Antioquia). During the time I spent at the CRL, the number of soldier-patients undergoing Glucantime treatment fluctuated between 50 and 120.

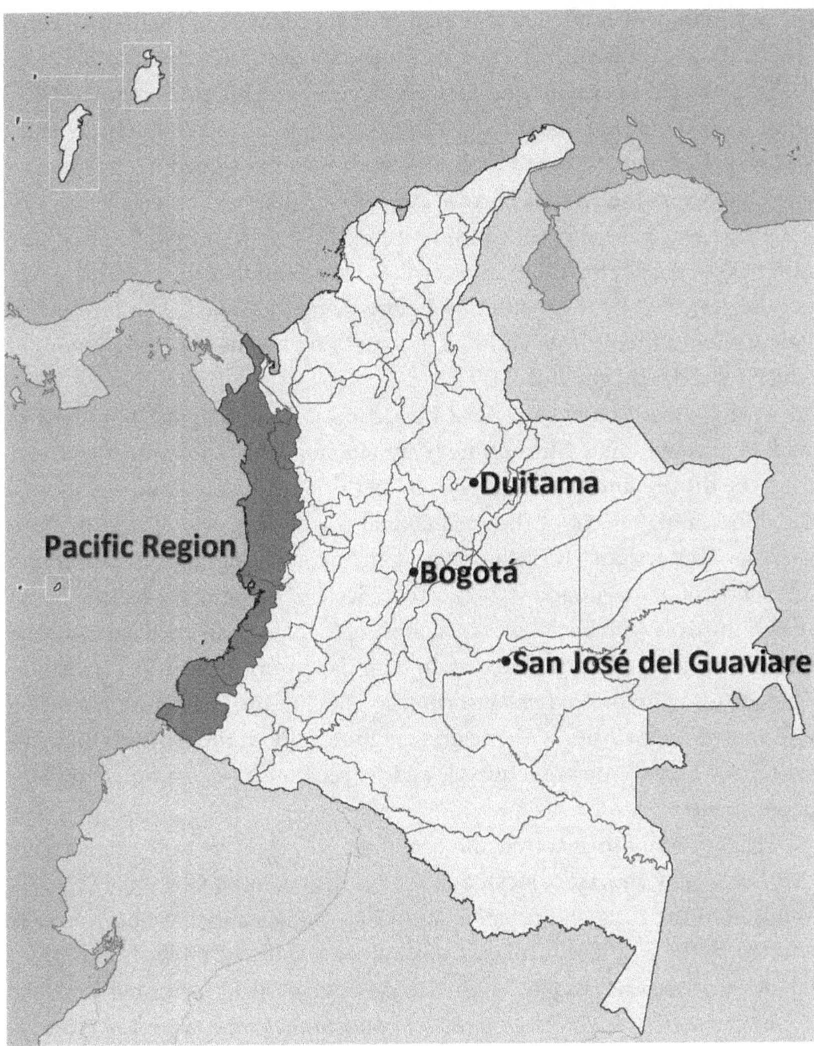

FIGURE I.2. Political map of Colombia indicating the capital, Bogotá, and the most important locations for fieldwork—the Pacific region and the cities of Duitama (Boyacá) and San José del Guaviare (Guaviare).

In a country that has been at war for more than fifty years, the Army is a large, extremely powerful, and rather impregnable institution, with some 250,000 members. As Ana María Forero Ángel reminds us, "The state of siege, of exception, and internal commotion was permanently declared in Colombia, which has resulted in the Army's stable enjoyment of exceptional powers" (2017, 46). Until that moment, my relationship with the Army and its members had been completely nonexistent. However, through family connections,

I was able to deliver a letter to a high-ranking member of the Public Force (Fuerza Pública) explaining who I was, what my research was about, and why I was interested in conducting part of my ethnographic project at the CRL. Since I was quite sure that my request was going to be categorically denied, I was surprised and excited to receive an authorization signed by the General Commander of the Armed Forces. The Public Force and especially the Colombian Army have always been very respectful toward my work. They have never asked me for anything in return or demanded that the research products be reviewed by the institution before being published. The intellectual independence I have been afforded is something I want to highlight and for which I feel deeply grateful.

At the CRL, I had the unique opportunity to accompany hundreds of soldiers through their Glucantime treatment and their subsequent recovery from the disease and the drug. I observed these young men putting up with the intoxicating effects of the medicine and grappling with their stubborn leishmaniasis lesions, while immersed in the daily dramas, humiliations, jokes, boredom, negotiations, and camaraderie of the military regime. I also shared my time with health workers, most of them women and civilians, who blended military and care practices in their daily work. Male officers responsible for disciplining soldiers and running most of the CRL's administration also shared their stories with me and taught me about the Army as an institution, how the center functioned, and its relationship with other military departments.

My research also involved three months of fieldwork in a municipality that I will call Candelario, located in the Pacific region of Colombia (fig. I.2). While both the rural and urban areas of this municipality have been heavily affected by the war, leishmaniasis constitutes a significant public health problem for Candelario's rurality. A biomedical research institution that I call the Leishmaniasis Research Institute (LERI), whose offices and laboratories are located in one of Colombia's largest cities, established a small permanent clinical facility in the urban area of Candelario in the 1980s. I am keeping the name of this research center and its locations anonymous because I do not wish to particularize institutional or personal responsibilities or disrupt valuable scientific projects and training currently taking place there. My aim is to discuss patterns that I know are not exclusive to LERI but shared by other institutions doing biomedical research on leishmaniasis in Colombia. Leishmaniasis patients from remote and impoverished rural areas of Candelario and nearby municipalities come to LERI to be diagnosed and treated. In turn, they enroll in clinical and other research studies. At LERI's facility in Candelario, I talked to several civilian patients affected by the disease, as well as the staff who recruit patients for internationally and nationally funded research projects on leishmaniasis. The regular paperwork, biomedical practices, and interactions with patients that develop within this small clinical facility, all of which enable the research LERI conducts, were of particular interest to my ethnographic exploration. Two scientific conferences—one national and one international—offered me further opportunities to learn about biomedical research on leishmaniasis and trace discourses, and to map additional actors involved in understanding and dealing with leishmaniasis in Colombia and elsewhere.

The clinical facilities where I conducted fieldwork—the CRL and LERI's facility in Candelario—are exceptional spaces for the medical management of leishmaniasis. There, both the concentration of leishmaniasis cases and the broad access people have to antileishmanial drugs are atypical. Nonetheless, at these special locations, the intersection of war and disease appears in ways that are both blatant and ordinary. "The sometimes uncanny ordinariness of such seemingly extraordinary circumstances" (Wool 2015, 3) is what allowed me to trace the pervasive expansion of violence and the daily maintenance of inequalities for leishmaniasis sufferers both within and outside of these sites.

By the time I began to conceive this project, it was clear that the voices of (ex-) guerrilla combatants had to be included in my work. Although I contacted people working for the state institution in charge of guerrilla members' processes of demobilization and reintegration into civilian life, authorization to conduct interviews with ex-combatants was a long and still uncertain process. While on vacation in Cuba in August 2016, just a month before returning to Colombia to start field research, I unexpectedly ended up at the hotel where the peace negotiations between the government and the FARC had been taking place since November 2012. There, I met Francisco, a midrank guerrilla commander who had been with the FARC for twenty-eight years. I felt tremendously fortunate when he told me by phone some days after our conversation at the hotel that a meeting could be arranged in Colombia with FARC members to discuss their experiences with leishmaniasis. That meeting occurred six months later, in February 2017, three months after the peace deal was signed.

During the early days of the implementation of the peace deal, which started on December 1, 2016, twenty-six so-called Transitional Zones for Normalization (Zonas Veredales Transitorias de Normalización, henceforth ZVNT) were established in rural areas of Colombia as part of the transition process for FARC members to congregate for a period of months and lay down arms. Two of these disarmament camps—Colinas and Charras—were located in Guaviare, a *departamento* in the south-central region of Colombia, the capital of which is San José del Guaviare (fig. I.2). In February 2017, I spent one week at the Colinas ZVNT, where approximately five hundred combatants had gathered, most of them from the legendary FARC Eastern Bloc (see *Verdad Abierta*, 2013). I discussed leishmaniasis with high-, mid-, and low-rank guerrillas and spent most of my time accompanying empirical nurses who had medical responsibilities within this guerrilla organization.

I conducted more than seventy semistructured interviews with a diverse group of actors: soldiers, subofficers, and officers of the Army, FARC guerrilla members, scientists, research staff, medical professionals, nursing assistants, peasants, fishers, woodcutters, representatives of multilateral health institutions, civil servants, and kidnapping survivors. As I listened to these people, my emotions included empathy, compassion, admiration, and hope—but also disdain, disagreement, resentment, and despair. I laughed and cried with them. Sometimes I celebrated their stories. At times, when I felt it was safe and I was given the space, I was able to amicably challenge their arguments and contrast them with my viewpoint. At other times, I intentionally avoided overhearing or participating in certain conversations. Occasionally, I opted for timid nodding or even silence.

As I conducted participant observation and interviews, there were only a few times when I felt like I was listening to rehearsed stories or prepared narratives; for example, in interviews with some public servants or high-ranking members of the Army. This is likely because talking about a health issue such as leishmaniasis does not seem to refer directly to violence or is perceived to be less fraught with political tensions. For the most part, however, my approach of viewing the armed conflict through stories about this disease prompted people to see themselves as victims of other types of violence generated by war or to recognize that war is experienced in ways other than those usually described. I realized that by delving into the dynamics of the conflict from an unusual vantage point such as leishmaniasis, it becomes more difficult to succumb to the narrative tropes that account for the Colombian armed conflict through the "traditional" places, mechanisms, and actors of the war. By adopting this *oblique* perspective, it becomes easier to account for the ubiquitous, inescapable, and penetrating nature of war expressed in realities that still remain largely unexplored. As noted by Michael Jackson, "In every human society, the range of experiences that are socially acknowledged and named is always much narrower than the range of experiences that people actually have" (2002, 23). This book demonstrates how narratives with atypical entry points—like leishmaniasis—"push back and pluralise our horizons of knowledge" about the war (2002, 25).

Chapter Outline

Each chapter of this book explores the *maraña* from a different point of view. My intention has been to pull and tighten some of its central threads to take a closer look at the elements that make up the *maraña* and the relationships that sustain it.

In chapter 1, "Leishmaniasis: A War Disease," I explore the ecological attachments of leishmaniasis-transmitting sandflies and the Colombian armed conflict as well as the war geographies of Colombian leishmaniasis. I show that leishmaniasis is one of the ways in which war alters people's lives by exposing them to vector bites, resulting in stigmatizing skin ulcers that can turn a benign disease lethal. I also attend to how war has altered the distribution and epidemiology of the disease itself, something scientists discuss but do not write about.

In chapter 2, "The Pharmaceuticalization of War," I follow the standard drug used to treat leishmaniasis along the legal and extralegal circuits through which it circulates. These trajectories allow me to unveil the discourses and practices that sustain the political economy of this drug and the social fragmentations of war that it reproduces.

In chapter 3, "Leishmaniasis within the Colombian Army," I explore the historical and political context whereby leishmaniasis became a strategic and security problem for the Army in its fight against insurgent groups. Tracing the measures adopted by this institution to face this problem and ensure the continuity of the war, I uncover the therapeutic machinery to return soldiers to service but not to health.

In chapter 4, "Glucantime and the Politics of Cure," I dwell on the bodily experience of the soldier with leishmaniasis as he undergoes one or more treatments for the disease. Attentive to his physical and emotional deterioration throughout this process, I show that the privileged access soldiers have had to antileishmanial drugs is also deeply fraught with violence.

In chapter 5, "Pacified Scientific Accounts on Leishmaniasis," my interest focuses on the contradictions involved in understanding leishmaniasis in the midst of war and writing about this disease as if the conflict did not exist. I discuss how the pharmaceuticalization of biomedical research on neglected tropical diseases plays a central role in creating this paradox.

The conclusion of the book is a reflection on the violence that continues in Colombia despite the signing of a peace agreement. Thinking through *desenmarañamiento* and having peace on the horizon, I propose some actions that could lead to the disarming of the leishmaniasis experience in Colombia.

1

Leishmaniasis: A War Disease

As the Colombian war has mainly taken place within the forests where leishmaniasis-transmitting sandflies thrive, the disease has been especially harsh on combatants of the armed conflict—not only Army soldiers but also members of guerrilla and paramilitary groups. However, leishmaniasis similarly affects civilian populations who are involved in activities that take place within the jungle. These activities encompass legal ventures as well as war-intertwined illicit economies—for instance, cocaine production and illegal mining—that remain confined and hidden deep inside these forested environments. Thus, peasants, Indigenous peoples, *raspachines* (coca harvest workers), hunters, loggers, and miners whose daily activities are carried out in a close relationship with the tropical forests may also suffer from leishmaniasis. The same goes for any other person who, for one reason or another, approaches or enters the jungle, including tourists, photographers, biologists, and anthropologists.

Visible marks on the body, mostly painless skin sores that grow slowly and resist healing, are a distinctive characteristic of leishmaniasis and the primary physical manifestation of the disease. When they heal, these ulcers turn into scars—permanent evidence that someone has entered the jungle at least once, was bitten by a sandfly, and ended up infected with the parasite. Although guerrillas are far from the only population in Colombia who bear these skin lesions and their long-lasting marks, many still consider leishmaniasis to be the guerrilla disease.[1] As I show in this chapter, this label has been tremendously harmful because, in the Colombian context, being called a guerrilla member or guerrilla collaborator is virtually a death sentence. In the political arena, left-wing leaders are often branded as guerrillas, (narco)terrorists, or *castrochavistas*,[2] especially by former president Álvaro Uribe and members of his right-wing party. However, such accusations also affect civil society and pose serious and even life-threatening risks to FARC ex-combatants, social leaders, activists, human rights defenders, journalists, scholars, political and opinion leaders, humanitarian organizations' employees, or anyone who opposes the social order that perpetuates inequality and violence (LeGrand, van Isschot, and Riaño-Alcalá 2017). Being called *guerrillero* or *guerrillera* is one of the most dangerous accusations someone can receive. This label is perhaps the worst stigma a person can carry in contemporary Colombia.

Here, I draw on Omar Dewachi's work (2019) to examine the armed conflict as an ecology that generates the necessary conditions for the establishment of pathological relationships between microorganisms and humans. Focusing on an antibiotic-resistant bacterium that US military surgeons called *Iraqibacter*, Dewachi explores the biological and morbid legacies of war in the Middle East region. He challenges this moniker's racial connotations by asking what might be particularly Iraqi about this microorganism. He posits that *Iraqibacter* is a pathology of intervention that marks the culmination of decades of Western military actions in Iraq, which have altered the very ecosystem in which human and nonhuman life develops and forms relationships. Building on Dewachi's analysis, I demonstrate in this chapter that leishmaniasis constitutes one of the ways in which the armed conflict alters the lives of combatants and civilians in rural areas. Therefore, rather than a guerrilla disease, leishmaniasis should be considered *a war disease* in Colombia. This understanding comes to light in three main phenomena.

First, the war has funneled various parts of the population into the forest—mostly soldiers, guerrillas, paramilitaries, victims of kidnapping, victims of forced displacement, and coca growers and harvesters who consequently end up suffering from leishmaniasis ulcers and bearing leishmaniasis scars. Thus, the conflict is the driving force that leads them to become absorbed into the *maraña* and makes them vulnerable to sandfly bites and *Leishmania* infections. Second, through the constant movement of these people across, in, and out of the jungle, the war has also caused leishmaniasis to move to places and emerge in areas where there had never been cases before. In other words, the epidemiological behavior of the disease has been critically reshaped by the armed conflict. Third, the stigmatization of leishmaniasis sufferers as guerrilla members is another significant way in which people experience the war by way of this disease. The perverse association between leishmaniasis and membership in a guerrilla group has engendered marginalization, discrimination, exclusion, and violence against guerrillas but also—and not incidentally or collaterally—against civilians affected by leishmaniasis.

My understanding of leishmaniasis-related stigma and discrimination begins at the very place and materiality where ulcers take shape—the skin. As the body's largest organ, the skin contains and protects us from the world but also exposes us to others (Ahmed and Stacey 2001). Skin has the ability to register both the passage of time and particular events in our biographies. "Skin remembers both literally in its material surface and metaphorically in resignifying on this surface, not only sex, race and age, but the quite detailed specificities of life histories" (Prosser 2001, 52). Although it is a highly imprecise historical record, we ask the skin to tell us something about the person it covers, to give away information about their identity, to reveal a hidden truth, or to give us access to a cloaked past (Prosser 2001). As a contact surface through which bodies are exposed to bodies, the skin "cannot refuse an impression" (Segal 2009, 44). People can't skin themselves, no matter how much they want to. The skin is always open to a reading and cannot but answer questions about the subject who wears it. Yet the ways in which the skin comes to matter are always subject to a particular time and place (Ahmed and Stacey 2001). This chapter shows how, in the context of the Colombian armed conflict, leishmaniasis ulcers locate the jungle on people's skin and are exposed to a reading through the lens of war. Skin marked by the jungle becomes invested with the cultural burdens of armed violence. Through this skin geography (Adams-Hutcheson 2017), the jungle is preserved in the most visible part of the body, and a cutaneous referent (a leishmaniasis ulcer or scar) and the social inferiority of the subject (demonized guerrilla fighter) become inseparable and stigmatizing.

My analysis also draws on the conceptual framework of stigma developed by Richard Parker and Peter Aggleton (2003) in the case of HIV/AIDS. These authors argue that taking Goffman's classic work (1986) as a starting point has led to ineffective and problematic ways of understanding and, consequently, researching and addressing stigma. In their view, defining stigma "as something *in* the person stigmatized, rather than as a designation that others attach *to* that individual" (R. Parker and Aggleton 2003, 15) results in an individualistic interpretation of the problem. Thus, studies and interventions taking this approach end up focusing on the beliefs and attitudes of those who stigmatize and on the emotional responses of stigmatized individuals. Moreover, the research that builds on Goffman's work tends to assume that stigmatization would disappear if stigmatizers were given access to the "right" information and if stigmatized individuals were equipped with skills to better cope with the effects of stigmatization. Parker and Aggleton challenge this sort of understanding and approach. For them, stigma and discrimination "are social and cultural phenomena linked to the actions of whole groups of people, and are not simply the consequences of individual behavior" (2003, 17). In their view, making sense of stigma requires paying attention to the structural dimensions of discrimination that use stigmatization to produce and reproduce social inequality and exclusion. Based on this understanding, in this chapter, I examine the societal and historical dynamics that led to the establishment of a harmful association between leishmaniasis and guerrilla groups, resulting in tragic consequences not only for guerrillas with this disease but also for civilians whose lives have been similarly but not equally *enmarañados* with the jungle and the armed conflict.

Leishmaniasis Is More Jungle

"There is no peace in the jungle," wrote Luis Eladio Pérez in a memoir about his seven years as a hostage of the FARC (2008, 73). He was referring not only to the inescapable noises and liveliness of this place but also to the distinctive location of war in Colombia (Ospina 2014). Although the armed conflict comprises a myriad of phenomena that have manifested in many different scenarios and landscapes throughout the country, the jungle is the emblematic space where the war has been fought. Since colonial times, imperial-, state-, and nation-building projects have persistently failed at incorporating the vast amounts of land on either side of the three mountain chains that cross the center of the country diagonally from south to north. These extensive geographies correspond to more than half of Colombia's present-day national territory. For reasons ranging from the organization of resistance blocks by peasant, Indigenous, or Afro communities to very challenging access conditions, difficult climates, and natural settings deemed untamable, the jungles have remained peripheral and are still considered an inversion of civic and social order (Serje 2014).

According to conventional wisdom in Colombia, jungles are regarded as diseased, remote, and problematic lands; immersed in violence; occupied by marginal people engaged in illegal activities; and in need of order, development, and modernization (Serje 2005). Due to the protracted armed conflict, these spaces are still known today as "red zones," or *zonas de orden público* (public order areas)—war zones where different armed actors dispute the territorial control over areas considered strategic for cocaine production and trafficking, gold mining, oil exploitation, palm oil plantations, and other types of legal or illegal extractive activities (see Molano Bravo, 2005). It is thus important to understand that while the space of the Colombian armed conflict is not limited to the physical boundaries of the forests, on a discursive, symbolic, material, and experiential level, it remains the primary setting in which war unfolds (Cárdenas and Duarte Torres 2016).

The boundaries of the jungle also delimit the ecologies to which leishmaniasis-transmitting sandflies belong. These insects are tiny and hairy, with body lengths ranging from 1.5 to 4 mm. Their wings are large compared to their minute bodies. The whitish color of these little creatures is probably the reason why people in Colombia commonly call them *manta blanca* (white blanket), or *manta*, for short. During my fieldwork, I heard people referring to sandflies as *manta*, *manta blanca*, or *palomilla*. However, I have found documents where names such as *aliblanco*, *jején*, *capotillo*, *arenilla*, and *pringador* also appear. The rainforest offers all kinds of shelter for these animals to spend most of the day. When the sun sets, females take an active flight near the ground in search of mammalian blood to nourish their eggs. The war has constantly funneled various human groups into the jungle and made them stay there for long periods, turning them into easily available prey for sandflies and vulnerable to *Leishmania* infections. As such, the conflict is a powerful force that pulls people into the *maraña*, leading to human-nonhuman interactions of a pathological nature.

Among the 31,283 victims of kidnapping between 1958 and June 2023 (Observatorio de Memoria y Conflicto 2023), Ingrid Betancourt remains the most famous survivor. In 2002, when she was campaigning for the presidency of Colombia, she and her campaign manager Clara Rojas were held captive by the FARC for six years of inhumane cruelty. Due to her dual Colombian-French citizenship and high political profile, Ingrid Betancourt's kidnapping received worldwide media coverage. It became a diplomatic priority for the then-presidents of Colombia, Venezuela, and France: Álvaro Uribe, Hugo Chávez, and Nicolas Sarkozy, respectively. In the memoir she published in 2010 about the tragic years she was forced to spend in the jungle, she wrote this about one of her experiences with sandflies:

> That night another plague lay in wait: the *manta blanca*. It covered us like snow, spreading over our clothes and into our skin, inflicting painful bites that we could not avoid. *La manta blanca* was a compact cloud of microscopic pearl-colored midges with diaphanous wings. It was hard to believe that these fragile things, so clumsy in flight, could inflict such painful bites. I tried to kill them with my hands, but they were insensitive to my efforts, because they were so tiny and light that it was impossible to crush them against my skin. We had to retreat and take the path to the river earlier than planned. We plunged with relief into its warm water, scratching our faces with our nails to free ourselves from the last relentless insects chasing us. (Betancourt 2010, 405)

Ingrid Betancourt does not seem to relate her encounters with sandflies with the leishmaniasis outbreaks she witnessed among guerrillas and other kidnapping victims while she was held captive. But, for Luis Carlos, a seasoned FARC member I interviewed in the disarmament camp of Colinas, the memory of his first experience with leishmaniasis *is* a story about sandflies. He joined this guerrilla group almost thirty years before we met. Luis Carlos was a town council member affiliated with the Unión Patriótica (UP), a political party founded in 1984 by the FARC as agreed on in the negotiations between this guerrilla group and the government of Belisario Betancur (1982–1986). Since the foundation of the UP, many of its members and sympathizers have become victims of kidnapping, forced disappearance, and assassinations. This tragic phenomenon, known as "the genocide of the UP," resulted in the murder or forced disappearance of 5,733 people between 1984 and 2016, according to figures published in 2022 by the Special Jurisdiction for Peace (JEP). Intending to save his life, Luis Carlos joined the ranks of the FARC. Within this organization, he served as commander of different guerrilla *columnas* in central and southern Colombia. He was also the founder of a FARC radio station, part of the FARC team behind the peace talks during the government of Andrés Pastrana (1998–2002), and involved in the negotiations in Havana that culminated in a successful peace agreement in 2016. This is how Luis Carlos recalled his first encounter with leishmaniasis:

> Let's see. I got to know leishmaniasis between 1992 and 1993, on the Unilla River [located in Guaviare] . . . I remember very well that we were on the river and we had to sail for an hour with a canoe to cut wood. In the morning, we were dropped in certain area to cut a type of green firewood that's called *bizcocho*, which fires when it's green and does not smoke.[3] . . . In that part of the rainforest, there was *manta blanca*, as we call the little mosquito. You would lift the leaves with your fingers and you could find the insects there, during the day, orbiting [pointing upward, he made a circular gesture with his finger]. I was cutting wood with an axe. I was sent there when there were already several cases of leishmaniasis in the camp. Indeed! A few days later I had a leishmaniasis sore on my hand!

Because of the strong ecological attachments between sandflies and the jungle, leishmaniasis is virtually limited to this space. Unlike other diseases that also occur in this environment, leishmaniasis is almost exclusively a jungle disease. For scientists, the so-called dogma of leishmaniasis on the American continent is rooted in the viewpoint that this disease is a zoonosis with a sylvatic transmission cycle. In other words, leishmaniasis is understood as a disease transmitted by sandflies from wild animals to humans, with the life cycle of the *Leishmania* parasite primarily depending on the sandflies' access to jungle mammals that serve as their standard blood source. When a sandfly bites an infected wild mammal and then bites a human, the human becomes infected with the *Leishmania* parasite and might develop an ulcer. Under that dogmatic view, wild animals are absolutely necessary for human infection to take place, and humans are just accidental hosts who become infected with the parasite when they enter the forest.

The spatial entanglement of leishmaniasis and the jungle provides such a significant part of the medical understanding of the disease that health workers tend to rule out leishmaniasis if the consulting patient denies having recently been in this setting. In fact, contact with the forest is regularly considered a condition for proceeding with the diagnosis of the disease (MinSalud and INS 2017, 9). On occasions, this principle means that some people do not even get to see a doctor when their sores do not seem to have emerged from the jungle. I had the opportunity to witness this logic in action at LERI's clinical facility, located in the urban area of Candelario. One morning, a lady in her fifties or sixties knocked on the clinic's door. Ramiro, one of the nursing assistants, opened the door halfway and, without letting her in, asked what she wanted. She asked him if that was the place where people get treated against *guaral*, as leishmaniasis is popularly called in that area of Colombia. Ramiro asked her if she was the one with the sore. She replied that it wasn't her but her father. Before bringing him in, she expressed that she had preferred to come alone and find out if this clinic was the right place. "Where is he from?" Ramiro asked. "From here, from Candelario," she replied. "Here in Candelario [referring to the urban area] there is no *guaral*. What your dad has is not *guaral*." He said these words as he slammed the door in her face. Thus, the lady's father was not even given the opportunity to see the doctor because his case was prematurely dismissed on the grounds of not being connected to the jungle.

In interviews with scientists, public health officials, and health professionals, I asked about the particularities of leishmaniasis, about those characteristics that make this disease different from other illnesses also transmitted by insect vectors, such as Chagas disease or malaria. I was repeatedly told that, although Chagas disease also affected poor people in rural areas of Colombia, the domestic space is the principal place of encounter between humans and the triatomine bugs that transmit Chagas—particularly in precariously built houses with adobe walls or thatched roofs, where these insects like to live. Therefore, unlike leishmaniasis, Chagas was definitely not a jungle disease.

Establishing a spatially based differentiation between malaria and leishmaniasis was slightly more complicated. However, Adriana Nieto helped me understand the geographical peculiarities of each disease. Adriana is a microbiologist specializing in epidemiology, and she has worked for sixteen years leading the public health institution in charge of vector-borne diseases in Candelario. The rural area of this municipality has been profoundly affected not only by leishmaniasis and the armed conflict but also by malaria. As Candelario is often among the five municipalities reporting the majority of malaria cases in Colombia, controlling malaria is the absolute priority of Adriana's institution. Based on her extensive experience with both diseases, Adriana described the main difference between them as follows: "Leishmaniasis is more jungle; the disease is really *selvática* [from the jungle]. Instead, malaria has both peri-urban transmission and transmission in rural areas. We can say it is not so *selvática*. While leishmaniasis is clearly *selvática*, malaria is in both places, but primarily in areas a little bit more populated by people. . . . In malaria's case, *we* are the parasite's reservoir, and *we* carry the parasite with us . . . because the reservoir is the human. For leishmaniasis, the reservoir is not the human but the animal that is in the jungle."

Anopheles mosquitoes transmitting malaria do not inhabit only the jungle. They are often found in urban and peri-urban areas, living with humans in or around houses (Montoya-Lerma et al. 2011). Moreover, malaria is considered an anthroponosis, which means that humans are sources of infection and the disease can be transmitted by the mosquito from human to human, without the need for a mediating mammal or bird. While this can also be true for leishmaniasis, sandflies are primarily jungle beings, insects that need the humid and forested ecologies of the jungle to survive, even in the few cases when they spend part of their lives around and within rural houses (Ocampo et al. 2012). Leishmaniasis on the American continent is generally regarded as a zoonotic disease; that is, an illness that is transmitted by sandflies that feed on infected jungle mammals. While transmission from human to human (anthroponotic transmission) is plausible and a matter of scientific debate (Ferro et al. 2015; Martínez-Valencia et al. 2017; Vergel et al. 2006), scientists agree that the predominant transmission cycle of leishmaniasis takes place within the forest.

It is the spatial encounter between the multiple species involved in leishmaniasis, the complex phenomenon of the armed conflict, and the metamorphic ecologies of the jungle that have contributed to making this disease an illness of war in Colombia. They all belong to the *maraña* that holds leishmaniasis and the conflict together. Arturo Casas, a FARC nurse who joined the guerrilla group in 1998, shares the same interpretation. Only one year after his recruitment, he was trained as a guerrilla nurse through an eleven-month medical course periodically offered to a few members of the organization. Although he was already familiar with this disease from having previously worked as a peasant and *raspachín*, it was during this training that he heard the word *leishmaniasis* for the first time. Since joining the FARC, he had to deal with countless leishmaniasis cases within the guerrilla ranks.

When I asked him to describe the relationship between the disease and the war, he used the following words: “Leishmaniasis and the armed conflict are connected through the conditions in which *la lucha* [the fight or the struggle] takes place. If *la lucha* was urban, there would be no leishmaniasis. But *la lucha* is rural; it is in the jungle.” Both leishmaniasis and the war take place far away from the Colombian urban centers, far away from the cities. It is also in these peripheral and rural areas where people have struggled the most to defend dignified ways of living that run counter to modernizing ideas and development projects brought by extractive corporations, political elites, and the central government. Leishmaniasis happens in places where armed and social conflict has traditionally occurred. Since the jungle provides the setting for war, and leishmaniasis is the disease of the jungle, leishmaniasis has acquired a powerful meaning as a disease of war in Colombia. As the jungle has become a *war ecology* in Colombia (Dewachi 2019), leishmaniasis has become a disease of the war in this context.

The War Geographies of Leishmaniasis

“What do you think is particular about Colombian leishmaniasis? What happens here that doesn’t happen elsewhere?” I posed this question to Cristian Ortega, a veterinarian who has worked on leishmaniasis research for more than thirty years, most of which he spent studying how multiple species participate in the transmission of this disease in Colombia. He explained to me that, unlike other places, the epidemiology of leishmaniasis in Colombia has clearly changed in relation to the armed conflict. “That’s something we’ve been commenting on for twenty years. And not only do we see it, other research groups have seen it as well,” he said. Cristian was specifically referring to the human migrations associated with the war and the resulting and unexpected emergence of leishmaniasis cases in places where this disease was rare or nonexistent before. “I think that Colombia differs from other contexts because the process of violence and the confrontations between the military and guerrilla groups cause changes in the different species of *Leishmania* in the country. It seems to me that this does not happen in other countries. I mean, generally speaking, the same species of *Leishmania* stays in the same place, it doesn’t move as it happens here in Colombia.” Cristian mentioned the case of Chaparral as a good example of what he meant by this. Between 2003 and 2006, the largest leishmaniasis outbreak documented in Colombia took place in Chaparral—a town of nearly sixty thousand people located in the south of Tolima. While the number of reported cases in Tolima until 2002 had been traditionally low (840 cases in the 1980s and 1,833 cases in the

1990s), 2,313 cases were reported in five years (2003–2007) alone in Chaparral (Valderrama-Ardila et al. 2010; Pardo et al. 2006). The town hospital went from seeing a few sporadic leishmaniasis cases in 2002 to suddenly diagnosing, reporting, and treating an overwhelming number of patients in 2003 and the subsequent years of that epidemic event (see also Santaella et al. 2011). Since that unprecedented outbreak, Chaparral became an endemic municipality for leishmaniasis—a place where the disease is regularly found among people living in that area.

Scientists studying leishmaniasis in research institutions located in the major Colombian urban centers—Bogotá, Cali, and Medellín—recognized in the Chaparral epidemic an important opportunity for research. One of the studies showed that the most probable parasite species responsible for the outbreak was *Leishmania (V.) guyanensis* (Rodríguez-Barraquer et al. 2008). Until that moment, this species had only been reported in the southeastern region of Colombia, in the Amazon River basin. Therefore, scientists were surprised to confirm the presence of *L. (V.) guyanensis* in a very different location, "strikingly different from the primary tropical rain forests of lower altitudes" to which this parasite species was believed to be confined (Rodríguez-Barraquer et al. 2008, 279). Another article went further, claiming that "in the Chaparral outbreak, the dominant parasite species was *Leishmania (V.) guyanensis*, and its novel occurrence suggested that the origin of the outbreak may have been caused by the movement of persons, possibly including armed groups, from the Amazon or Orinoco basin" (Valderrama-Ardila et al. 2010, 248).

Cristian explained what happened in Chaparral:

> Several things came together. Fundamentally, there was a susceptible population for which leishmaniasis did not exist before, at least not significantly. There was also a species, *Leishmania guyanensis*, which was not in that area before. Then, someone brought that *guyanensis* there. One of the things that people used to say is that that area was a resting place for the guerrillas. Then, those infected guerrillas served as reservoirs, as sources of parasites that enable for a cycle of leishmaniasis transmission to get established there . . . The [insect] vector was taking parasites from one human and passing them on to another.

More than a "resting place for guerrillas," armed actors have traditionally been present in Chaparral and its neighboring municipalities in southern Tolima. In fact, the now-extinct FARC guerrilla movement was founded by 'Manuel Marulanda Vélez' in that area in 1964 (CNMH 2014). Guerrilla organizations and paramilitaries, as well as drug trafficking and the production of the opium poppy, have left a historical legacy of violence in that region. In the late 1990s and early 2000s, the FARC "used to move large troop contingents; in a single march they could move up to a thousand guerrillas" (Avila 2019, 296), which might explain the movement of *L. (V.) guyanensis* from the Amazon to Tolima. Moreover, in the late 1990s, Tolima was one of the areas where the FARC exercised strong social and territorial control. Thus, with the Democratic Security Policy of Álvaro Uribe's government, several Army operations focused on the south of Tolima (Fundación Ideas para la Paz 2013). This military offensive took place during the years of the leishmaniasis epidemic in Chaparral.

Adela Niño is a physician with doctoral training in parasitology and tropical medicine. She has worked for more than thirty years researching tropical diseases at a Colombian public university. Adela shares Cristian's interpretation of the way the disease has moved geographically. For her, the relationship between leishmaniasis and the war is most evident when studying the ways the epidemiological behavior of the disease has been shaped by the migratory movement of armed actors. As combatants have carried the parasite from one place to another, one can describe the bodily condition of the *Leishmania* infection as having leached into the environmental condition:

> One of the things we've seen is that, if you look at the map of the distribution of the different *Leishmania* species, there were areas where there wasn't a certain type of parasite, and then it appeared. One of the things we started to see in Valle del Cauca was that, when there were guerrilla movements in Dagua or the Cañón de Garrapatas, leishmaniasis foci began to appear among civilians where we had never had a record of that . . . I've seen the movement and appearance of leishmaniasis in areas where there was no leishmaniasis before. . . . The evidence, at least the epidemiological evidence, seems to show that, where there have been guerrilla movements, where they arrive, where they pass, leishmaniasis begins to appear. In other words, they come infected. They infect the insects [sandflies] that are located there and establish outbreaks. That is the hypothesis some of us have, but we have not tested it, it has not been tested.

Roberto Quintero is another physician who has devoted more than thirty-five years of his life to leishmaniasis research in Colombia, primarily studying the ecological factors leading to leishmaniasis transmission. I met him at the WorldLeish scientific conference in 2017, and some months after that, I visited Roberto's lab located at one of the main public universities in the country. Although Adela and Roberto have worked for different institutions and in different rural areas, Roberto told me the following story to describe the same sort of phenomenon Adela had observed:

> In 1986, in Montebello, Antioquia, two people from another region came to the *veredas* [hamlets] of Campoalegre and La Merced. Altogether, they had eleven active leishmaniasis lesions. Two months later, the first cases of leishmaniasis began to appear, and it quickly grew exponentially. . . . The relationship between those who arrived and the establishment of the outbreak was clear, and that is what you commonly hear when you talk to the community. [People say] "There was no such disease here, but the Army arrived, the guerrilla arrived, no matter who it was, they settled here and brought us the disease."

Even though Cristian, Adela, and Roberto were clear and frank in their accounts, no scientific article tells this story in such a straightforward way. Actually, in the papers that scientists publish, authors often refrain from mentioning the armed conflict and are extremely cautious about suggesting associations between the emergence of epidemiological events and the migration of military personnel, armed groups, and victims of forced displacement.[4] In other words, the conflict is often omitted from scientific accounts of leishmaniasis in Colombia or is barely named as one of the many social determinants that might be significant in the disease epidemiology (for instance, Herrera et al. 2018). Sometimes, the armed conflict is mentioned as a barrier in the execution of research projects but excluded as a possible explanation of the results (see Santaella et al. 2011).

This is likely due to the positivist approach used to understand and explain relationships between diseases and other phenomena, which, despite scientists' observations and intuitions, limits the type of claims they feel comfortable making. When I asked Cristian how he could *know* what he was telling me, he said: "No, you can't know, you can only guess, hypothesize." That is probably why he and many others have not explicitly written that war prominently shapes leishmaniasis's epidemiology in Colombia. Also, based solely on the data collected by the public health surveillance system, it would be very difficult—and sometimes ethically questionable—to study whether the occurrences of leishmaniasis cases are linked to events related to the armed conflict or whether the disease predominantly affects combatants other than those of the state military (i.e., members of guerrilla or paramilitary organizations) or people involved in conflict-related economies. While the report form used in the public health surveillance of leishmaniasis gathers information about the place where each case occurred, these data rely on, and are limited by, the information provided by the patient. Although this form collects information about the occupation of the patient, this information must be reported in the form of a code coming from a classification system of the

International Labour Organization (ILO). Of course, *guerrilla member, coca grower*, or *paramilitary* are not among the recognized categories.[5]

Despite this tendency to omit the conflict in scientific publications, several scientists I spoke with agreed that the war has played a fundamental role in shaping and altering leishmaniasis's geographic distribution. Many of them even consider that this particular association is the most characteristic aspect of Colombian leishmaniasis. If we consider these views and interpretations seriously, it becomes clear that war is central to the constitution and epidemiological behavior of leishmaniasis in Colombia today. It is then possible to argue not only that leishmaniasis and war are deeply *enmarañados* because they move alongside each other but also that the people who move leishmaniasis from one rural space to another are not alien to armed conflict. On the contrary, their lives are linked to the war in complex and diverse ways. Moreover, it becomes evident that the "natural" history of leishmaniasis cannot be told without considering the "human" history of war, making divisions between nature and culture seem highly inadequate. Thus, any account of this disease—epidemiological, biomedical, or otherwise—that takes the war into serious consideration will be better positioned to elucidate and address the contemporary reality of leishmaniasis in Colombia.

Drawing on Hannah Landecker's work on the *biology of history*, understood as the ways in which "human events and processes have materialized as biological events and processes and ecologies" (2016, 21), Omar Dewachi points to "the complex context of war and its contribution to the changing ecologies of antibiotic resistance" (2019, 10). He hypothesizes that the emergence of antibiotic-resistant bacteria in Iraqis' wounds and bodies may be no more than the biological legacy of a long history of war, which has led to critical circumstances such as the collapse of health care infrastructure and the constant movement of wounded patients—and bacteria—across the region. Similarly, the association between wartime migrations and the changes in *Leishmania* parasites' geographical distribution registers the footprints of war in the ecology and epidemiology of leishmaniasis in Colombia. That is, we might find a historical record of the armed conflict and associated human migrations in the changing spatial and temporal distribution of *Leishmania* parasites.

Michael Taussig has defined the *public secret* as "that which is generally known, but cannot be articulated" (1999, 5). When people are not able to say what they all know, he argues, power is at work. The absence of "hard facts" to prove or disprove the epidemiological association of war and leishmaniasis as well as the fear of uncertainty in science have downplayed how this disease and the armed conflict remain *enmarañados*. Also, acknowledging publicly that science does not take place in isolation from the war can be detrimental to researchers themselves. Under such circumstances, it may become difficult to obtain funding, ongoing research projects may be affected, and the work of scientists may be interpreted as "contaminated" by political issues. But perhaps we have reached a point where the lack of scientific evidence—in the traditional sense—should not stop us from articulating, writing, and discussing how important and central the war has been for leishmaniasis in Colombia. Moreover, the *maraña* formed by these two phenomena, as we will continue seeing in this and the following chapters, goes well beyond the epidemiological patterns of leishmaniasis. Thus, if we ever expect to be able to *desenmarañar* the war from the experience of leishmaniasis, as is the ultimate objective of my work, we need to start articulating the problem in a significantly more explicit and nuanced manner than what existing scholarship has produced so far (see Moore 2013). It is imperative that we probe beyond the current understandings of the epidemiological characteristics of leishmaniasis, even if this involves acknowledging, accepting, and also embracing messy uncertainty.[6]

The Guerrilla Disease

In my childhood, especially when we were on a road trip, my parents used to tell my sister and me that if we were ever stopped by men dressed in camouflage, we had to look at their feet to know if they were Army soldiers or guerrillas. If they were soldiers, they would be wearing leather boots. If they were guerrillas, they would be wearing rubber boots. This association between rubber boots and guerrillas has been circulated extensively in Colombia (García 1994; Molano Bravo 2001, 172). Since this bloody conflict has pitted Colombians against Colombians, it is difficult to tell in certain rural areas who is who and whether a person belongs, has affinities, or has been forced to relate to one side or another of the conflict. As Timothy P. Wickham-Crowley has noted, in guerrilla warfare, "the political enemy is no longer a foreign devil, but armed forces composed of one's own countrymen" (1992, 4). As such, arbitrary and discriminatory mechanisms have often emerged to distinguish between friends and foes.

Of course, it is not only guerrillas who wear rubber boots in Colombia. "They are also the boots used by the immense rural country, made up of peasant workers, farmers, *corteros* [sugar cane cutters], Indigenous peoples," and many others (V. Quintero 2009). Thus, the connotation attached to rubber boots has had violent and even deadly consequences for both civilians and guerrilla members at the hands of the Army and paramilitary groups (CINEP 2010; Ibañez Sarco 2015). The situation is so dramatic that some people in rural areas refuse to wear these boots for fear of being singled out as guerrillas (La Nación 2005; Ruta Pacífica de las Mujeres 2013).

Leishmaniasis has played a similar role in the Colombian conflict as rubber boots have. Although the disease and the marks it leaves on the body are not specific to members of guerrilla organizations, for many, leishmaniasis is a guerrilla illness. As such, this disease bears a double stigma in war-ridden Colombia. It involves not only the fleshy and visible body marks that characterize the disease but also the social stigma that establishes a perverse association with demonized guerrilla groups. The leishmaniasis-related stigma has contributed to deepening the degradation to which people belonging to guerrilla groups have been historically subjected in public discourse. The association between this illness and insurgent groups is nothing different than the cultural production of "negatively valued difference . . . as central to the establishment and maintenance of the social order" that originates in the rationales of the protracted armed conflict (R. Parker and Aggleton 2003, 17).

In my conversations with scientists and health professionals who have conducted leishmaniasis research for several years, all agreed that this disease is stigmatized as a guerrilla illness. Luciana Pérez, for example, is an epidemiologist who has been involved in research projects on infectious diseases for the past twenty years. During the last ten years, she has primarily focused on leishmaniasis. For her, a formulaic relationship has been maintained between leishmaniasis and subversive actors. In her words, the disease carries "a key punishing label: that Leishmaniasis = Guerrilla. And that label works here and in any corner of Colombia . . . Leishmaniasis = Guerrilla, that is one of the aspects that, in the last three or four decades, has characterized the disease in our country." For other health professionals involved in leishmaniasis research, however, the stigmatization of leishmaniasis patients is not equally widespread across the country. Adela Niño—one of the scientists I mentioned before—thinks that "the myth that leishmaniasis only affected guerrillas and those who got into the *monte* [forest]" circulates primarily in the cities, in central areas of the country, and also in places like Caquetá, Meta, and Putumayo where the FARC used to have a very strong presence. In her opinion, this stigmatizing notion is not as dominant in settings where leishmaniasis affects people who are clearly not directly involved in armed conflict—young children, for example. Based on her description of how the stigma works, the construction of leishmaniasis as a guerrilla disease has primarily operated in areas where the constitution of a social regime requires the constant reinforcing of guerrillas as inferior people in the public imagination. Thus, stigmatization does not occur uniformly throughout the national territory but is specific to conflict zones and spaces where the disease and, specifically, the marks it leaves on the skin needs to be attached to certain individuals and turned into a *homeland pathology* according to a war logic (Hochman, Liscia, and Palmer 2012). After all, "skin is a site of cultural inscription . . . [that] contains ideas about surfaces, boundaries, self and Other" (Adams-Hutcheson 2017, 3). Therefore, the stigmatization attached to leishmaniasis skin lesions should not be understood "as isolated phenomenon, or expressions of individual attitudes or of cultural values, but as central to the constitution of the social order" amid war (R. Parker and Aggleton 2003, 17).

This is consistent with how other forms of stigmatization have operated in the armed conflict context. In 2013, the National Center of Historical Memory (CNMH) published one of the most complete and groundbreaking reports documenting the phenomenon of being singled out and stigmatized as belonging to, collaborating with, or being an informant for one side or the other of the war, which has been an emblematic aspect of the Colombian armed conflict. Such stigmatization is described as "a process by which aspects such as marks on appearance, behavior, physical signs or place of residence are transformed into markers of belonging to the enemy's ranks and into a mechanism for blaming and pointing fingers at the civilian population" (CNMH 2013, 354). Not only individuals but entire populations were labeled as guerrillas or paramilitaries to justify the acts of persecution and extermination that followed. The CNMH showed that stigmatization became a widespread mechanism that took on local overtones based on how regional and local powers felt their interests were under threat. Thus, associating traits with guerrilla or paramilitary groups was a way to undermine political and civil rights at the local level, especially for individuals and organizations that promoted alternative and inclusive political, economic, and social systems.

Roberto Quintero—whom I previously mentioned—is convinced that the stigmatizing association between leishmaniasis and guerrillas has prevented people with ulcers from seeking medical help. Beatriz Rojas, one of his coworkers, shares this opinion. As a microbiologist with a postgraduate education in biomedical sciences, she has worked for almost thirty years investigating leishmaniasis in Colombia. According to Beatriz: "The truth is that many patients remain silent, thinking that they are going to be branded as guerrillas, right? In the case of an actual guerrilla member, the same thing happens because he thinks he's going to get arrested, right? And that's real, many people remain hidden or have remained hidden, suffering alone from the disease, or getting treated however they can, because of fear, because of that social stigma of being associated with one side or the other." Similarly, Luisa Álvarez, a nurse working for the Hospital San Juan Bautista in Chaparral, told me that in the rural areas of this municipality, "there were many civilians who complained that, if they went [to the health center] and showed that they had a sore in some part of their body, it was as if they were classifying themselves, self-proclaiming they were outlaws. They preferred to keep quiet, and use another type of medication such as herbs, plasters, multiple things, sometimes very drastic and very aggressive, and not go to see the doctor because there was so much taboo. Whoever had a sore suggestive of leishmaniasis was as if s/he were, in fact, a guerrilla member."

The FARC members I spoke with confirmed that the stigma linked to leishmaniasis had very real consequences for them during the war. Francisco, the FARC midrank commander who had facilitated my access to the disarmament camp in Colinas, brought up the story of "El Caleño" when I asked about the ways in which the stigmatization attached to leishmaniasis had affected members of this guerrilla organization. El Caleño was a young FARC member who had been infected with *Leishmania* in Medellín del Ariari (Meta) in 1991. Although he was given several injections of antileishmanial medication at the guerrilla camp, his skin lesion did not improve. At that time, Francisco said the FARC had not established systematic procedures to address the health problems affecting their troops. According to Julián Orjuela Benavides (2017, 50), this situation began to change around 1993, when FARC leaders decided at the VIII Guerrilla Conference to create a health policy for the insurgent organization, allocating a permanent budget for the health care of guerrilla members, the establishment of clandestine clinics, and the use of contraceptive implants. The commanders decided to take El Caleño out of the jungle and bring him to Bogotá to seek medical attention. However, he was arrested at the hospital. El Caleño spent almost five years in prison because of the connection drawn between his leishmaniasis marks and his guerrilla affiliation. "That was the way it was in the war," Francisco said. If a young man had leishmaniasis sores or marks on his body from military equipment, his cartridge belt, or boots, he would be detained. It was common for guerrillas with leishmaniasis to be arrested when they sought medical assistance. That is why FARC leaders eventually decided to forbid guerrilla members affected by leishmaniasis from leaving the jungle and approaching regular health care facilities.

The stigma attached to leishmaniasis and the state's part in creating this stigma are not exceptional or recent in Colombia's history. Diana Obregón (1996, 2002) has shown that the Colombian state and physicians played a decisive role in establishing a stigma around another disease—leprosy—which, like leishmaniasis, also leaves distinctive and visible marks on the body. At the turn of the twentieth century, physicians and scientists advocated for a bacteriological understanding and control of leprosy that, based on exaggerated figures and speeches loaded with repulsion for and aversion to the disease, materialized into severe and inhumane measures to segregate people with leprosy. The idea of leprosy as a highly contagious disease that inflicted inferior people, which emerged from the imperialist expansion of Europe and the United States, was embraced by Colombian physicians as a way to professionalize medicine in the country, establish a "national medicine," and be accepted into the European and North American scientific communities. Later, in the 1920s and 1930s, seeking Colombia's participation in the world market, physicians adopted a more relaxed attitude toward this disease to change the international perception that they themselves had created of Colombia as a leprosy nation. However, the cruel policies established for people with leprosy and their families still resonate with many Colombians for whom the name Agua de Dios—Colombia's most famous leprosarium—continues to be the title of a horror story (Platarrueda Vanegas 2008). Leishmaniasis is the heir to this historical legacy; it is even referred to as "the leprosy of the jungle" (see Betancourt 2010, 374; Emanuelsson 2012), a name that establishes a connection between the bodily marks and the social stigma that both illnesses involve, as well as the discriminatory effects on populations seen and constructed as inferior and deserving of misfortunes. After all, epidemics often serve to expose divisions within a society by revealing deep-seated power inequalities and antagonisms between social groups (Espinosa 2009).

Anthropologist Manuel Arias illustrates how the stigma of the guerrilla's disease has targeted not only FARC and other guerrilla combatants but also civilians who have been unfairly and dangerously singled out as guerrillas. As part of his fieldwork, Manuel accompanied a peasant organization in the highly conflictive Middle Magdalena region in 1998. During this time, he was diagnosed with malaria at the nearest health center in that rural area. Fortunately, treatment was accessible, and he recovered in just a few weeks. Two months later, he returned to the community to learn about the clandestine production of cocaine. To do so, he had to venture deep into the forest and stay for a week, hoping to understand each step of the process. Once back in Bogotá, he noticed two small sores on his hand and arm. Instead of healing with the use of ordinary disinfectants, his ulcers became bigger as time passed. Manuel then saw a general practitioner, who prescribed antibiotics, but the lesions continued to grow in both size and depth. Then he saw a dermatologist, who diagnosed leishmaniasis: "It's the famous *pito* that bit you, and that's what you have," she said. "But now, you need treatment, and that's where the problem begins." She told him to get a proper diagnosis—a biopsy—and ask the medical board of his health insurance company, called Saludcoop, to obtain Glucantime for him.

A month passed, the lesions got bigger, and Manuel still had no answer from Saludcoop about his medicine. Desperate, he talked to a Saludcoop nurse, who explained to him that this was "almost a political problem . . . because we all know that leishmaniasis only affects guerrillas." Enraged by these accusations, Manuel complained and even threatened to sue Saludcoop for slander and for not fulfilling its institutional mission. "I'm just one—among who-knows-how-many—suffering from leishmaniasis and if you don't give me the drug, I will sue," Manuel said to the nurse. After enduring more days without treatment and verbal accusations from Saludcoop's medical board that he was a guerrilla member, Manuel sought help from a relative who held the rank of Army colonel. When Manuel went through security at the Army's offices in Bogotá to see his relative, a lieutenant saw the bandage on his sores and asked: "What is that?" "A disease," Manuel replied. "That's leishmaniasis, isn't it?" "Yes, sir." "And why do you want to see my colonel?" "It's a family affair," Manuel replied. "*Guerrillero*, son of a bitch!" the lieutenant shouted and began to swear. Manuel's relative came out to see what was going on, and after scolding the lieutenant for the misunderstanding, he let Manuel in. Manuel's relative called the Federico Lleras Acosta Dermatological Center (a state research institute in Bogotá) to request health care and medication for Manuel. The next day, Manuel went to the center and received the Glucantime ampoules he needed for his treatment. The only condition in exchange for the drug was to return the empty ampoules to the institute every four days until he finished treatment as proof that he had not sold or given the medicine to anyone. As he reflected on this harrowing episode, Manuel told me: "Just imagine, a 23-year-old young man with leishmaniasis: he is a *guerrillero*, there's no way out of that . . . I began to reflect on what the actual consequences of this war are, and it really sucks. The story you hear that the problem is only forced displacement, deaths, murders. . . . Yes! Of course! But it's not only that. It's how the very everyday life gets fucked up. . . . War is lived from the smallest."

As the testimonies of Francisco and Manuel show, leishmaniasis ulcers and scars have been used to make certain distinctions among the Colombian population. In a guerrilla warfare context where anyone can be considered a potential enemy, the characteristic skin lesions of leishmaniasis have been used to differentiate—not unambiguously—between state enemies and civilians. The assumption here is that a person has leishmaniasis because they entered the jungle. And if that person entered the jungle, it is believed that they must be a guerrilla member, a guerrilla collaborator, or a participant in an illegal activity. In other words, a leishmaniasis sufferer is likely to be stigmatized as a criminal who deserves punishment from the state, a person against whom violence is not necessarily legal but always justified.

Paramilitary forces have followed the same rationale. This is evident in the testimonies of Jhon Jairo Esquivel Cuadrado (alias El Tigre) and Arnover Carvajal Quintana (alias Poca Lucha), two ex-members of the largest right-wing paramilitary group in Colombia: the United Self-Defenders of Colombia (AUC). As I mentioned earlier, the AUC was established in 1997 as an armed force to end leftist guerrilla movements and any expression of leftist ideology in Colombia. Álvaro Uribe's government launched a controversial demobilization process with the AUC coalition of paramilitary organizations in 2003, legally framed under Law No. 975 of 2005 and better known as the Law of Justice and Peace. These testimonies reveal that the detection of leishmaniasis lesions was explicitly part of the procedures used by paramilitaries to identify alleged guerrilla combatants and assassinate them.

El Tigre operated in Cesar in northeastern Colombia. He was found responsible for 13 massacres and 491 forced displacements as well as cases of rape, torture, kidnapping, and homicide and other crimes (*Verdad Abierta* 2010). Engelver García Pallares and Rafael Enrique Martínez Orozco were two of El Tigre's many murder victims. In the town of Codazzi (Cesar), Engelver and Rafael were widely known for selling fruits on the street. One day, very early in the morning, these two men were on their bikes looking for guavas on a farm on Verdecia Road. On their way back to Codazzi, they were stopped by two heavily armed men in an SUV who took them to an unknown place. These men were El Tigre and another AUC member known as Kevin. According to El Tigre, "alias 'Kevin' told him that they were not guava sellers but [guerrilla] militia, that one of them had been bitten by a *pito* [leishmaniasis], and that they were doing intelligence on the Army and the AUC" (*Verdad Abierta* 2009b; "Engelver García Pallares," n.d.). Based on this information, El Tigre ordered Kevin to kill Engelver and Rafael. The dead bodies were found next to two bicycles and four containers full of guavas. They were riddled with gunshot wounds.

Poca Lucha operated in Magdalena on the Caribbean Coast. He was directly involved in the murder of Simón Efraín González Ramírez on May 21, 2002, under the orders of José Gregorio Mangones Lugo (alias Carlos Tijeras), who was found to be responsible for this assassination as well as countless other crimes and human rights violations (*Verdad Abierta* 2009a). Simón was a twenty-two-year-old Colombian-French citizen who had traveled to Colombia to study at a university in Bogotá. Before beginning his classes, he decided to take a trip to the Sierra Nevada to practice meditation. On his way back, he was robbed and left with no money. While Simón was waiting for a truck that would take him closer to Bogotá, he was kidnapped and murdered by men in an SUV. His body was left in a banana waste dump in the municipality of Ciénaga (Magdalena). For Simón's parents, the tragedy did not end there. They faced multiple obstacles in recovering the body, as it had been buried as *NN* (John Doe) in a mass grave (*Verdad Abierta* 2011). According to Poca Lucha, the AUC's mission was "to combat common crime, our main enemy the guerrillas, their collaborators, muggers, *viciosos* [drug consumers], rapists and *jíbaros* [drug dealers]" (Avila Guarnizo 2010, 2). He also said that in order to identify their targets, paramilitaries often "look for [guerrilla] traces on people, such as boot traces, such as leishmaniasis, such as backpack or rifle marks on the shoulder." Poca Lucha suspects that Simón was likely subjected to this profiling, leading to the AUC's decision to kill him (Avila Guarnizo 2010, 5).

As I mentioned earlier, painless and growing skin lesions are the only physical manifestation of leishmaniasis. People can live with them—sometimes for weeks or even months or years—until the sores repel and disgust other people, until the discomfort affects labor and everyday activities, or until they heal. Leishmaniasis sufferers seek both home remedies and pharmaceutical treatments for their lesions to heal and turn into scars (Pinto-García 2025). As such, leishmaniasis is usually described by health professionals and scientists as a mostly benign, nondeadly disease. But, as the tragic stories of Engelver, Rafael, and Simón show, in the Colombian war context, leishmaniasis can also lead to violent death due to its deep stigmatization as a guerrilla disease. Hence, the protracted war has enabled the social construction of nondeadly leishmaniasis as a life-threatening disease to develop. The *enmarañamiento* of leishmaniasis and the war in Colombia has evolved in such a way that a seemingly harmless disease has become a death threat for not only guerrilla members. As a war disease, leishmaniasis affects people from all walks of life, not only restricting their access to medical and health services but also leading to their stigmatization, persecution, and death.

María Teresa Uribe de Hincapié explains that during the Cold War, a discourse on the dangers of communism made a profound impact in Colombia. Based on this narrative, governance strategies were established "that were not specifically aimed at defeating a guerrilla enemy—otherwise diffuse, confused with society, ambiguous, mobile—but rather to control alleged guerrillas' support bases represented in the rise of social movements" (Uribe de Hincapié 2001, 226). Indeed, the stigmatization of leishmaniasis—as well as the restrictions on access to leishmaniasis drugs, which I explore in the following chapter—harms not only guerrillas but also people living in rural areas who are exposed to the jungle for various reasons. These are people regarded by the state as a menace to development projects, modernizing plans, and the perpetuation of political elites in power. This should not be considered collateral damage; rather, these civilians are targeted and harmed by the cultural reading of the marks the jungle left on their skin—a skin geography mapped and *dermographed* by the armed and social conflicts (Ahmed and Stacey 2001, 15). With the guerrilla disease narrative constructed from the entanglement between leishmaniasis and the forests, this association and its sometimes fatal consequences have been mobilized as biopolitical weapons to damage this wider group of people in rural Colombia whom the state and paramilitary groups consider to be a threat to the political and social order.

Parker and Aggleton draw attention to the larger trajectories and power structures in which stigma and stigmatization are culturally produced: "It is vitally important to recognize that stigma arises and stigmatization takes shape in specific contexts of culture and power. Stigma always has a history which influences when it appears and the form it takes" (R. Parker and Aggleton 2003, 17). This approach requires us to challenge the notion of the guerrilla disease every time it is invoked. This is not only because of the devastating consequences this stigma involves but also because this language limits how we understand that the damage caused to civilians has not been simply incidental but part of a broader war logic that considers certain people threatening to the status quo. As Cynthia Enloe puts it: "If wounds and the wounded can be naturalized by sweeping them into the dismissive concept of 'collateral damage,' they won't matter" (Enloe 2023, 84). To make them matter is to disentangle the link between leishmaniasis and war by unraveling the threads of stigma and discrimination that bind those exposed to sandfly bites and *Leishmania* infections. This requires challenging the very structures of inequality and exclusion that have existed in Colombia for more than six decades—and which no peace agreement has the power to disintegrate.

2

The Pharmaceuticalization of War

The sun had risen a while ago. It was almost 6:30 a.m. on my first morning at the Transitional Zone for Normalization (ZVNT) in Colinas, where about five hundred members of the FARC had gathered after signing the agreement to lay down their arms. A month before my visit, in the last week of January 2017, the media had documented a major event in the history of Colombia. Complying with the terms of the peace deal signed in Havana, the FARC completed what was called *la gran marcha* (the great march): thousands of its members migrated from all corners of the national territory to the twenty-six zones—15 kilometers^2 in total—designated for their disarmament (Colombia2020 2017; *Semana* 2017).[1] The members of this guerrilla organization brought a few belongings, some animals, and the anxieties and hopes of a transition period marked by an unfinished war and a burgeoning peace. Working with the Colombian Army, UN representatives monitored this remarkable transit along rivers and highways; on foot; and in buses, vans, boats, and canoes. Images charged with symbolism, like those of guerrillas and soldiers exchanging smiles and shaking hands, filled many supporters of the peace deal with optimism.

While these encouraging scenes unfolded, however, the Army had not yet regained control of the territories that the FARC had abandoned, and other armed actors were already occupying them. In addition, the state had not been diligent in creating or adapting the necessary infrastructures in the ZVNTs so that FARC guerrillas could settle in those areas and prepare their reintegration process into civilian life (*Semana* 2017). These were some of the first signs of the government's noncompliance and lack of political will toward the implementation of what had been agreed on in Havana (see, for instance, *Verdad Abierta* 2017; Zamudio Palma 2017). During the administration of right-wing president Iván Duque (2018–2022), the FARC's situation became even more precarious and uncertain (Kroc Institute 2023). Since the signing of the peace agreement, 375 ex-FARC combatants and 1,514 social leaders and human rights defenders have been murdered (United Nations 2023; Avendaño Ladino 2023). Tragically, these figures continue to grow each month as I write this book.

When I arrived in Colinas at the end of February 2017, the ZVNT was far from ready or equipped for the guerrillas and their families to live there under adequate and dignified conditions. Notably, suitable living spaces were not yet available. Even though FARC members were still armed at the time of my visit (the FARC completed disarmament in June 2017), they had already begun their transition process to civilian life. During the day, about three hundred (ex-)combatants and one hundred civilians hired by the state worked hard on the construction of a small town. A few FARC commanders had carefully designed this village to meet the demands of a self-sufficient community inhabited by families who were supposed to live in separate houses while maintaining a strong sense of political unity and collective life beyond the end of the conflict (De Abreu 2017). In the meantime, (ex-)guerrillas were inhabiting makeshift huts made of wood poles, black plastics, and green tarp, which they had raised in a forested area of the ZVNT, protected from the sun by thick foliage (fig. 2.1). Although the leafy location and temporary appearance of these dwellings reminded me of wartime FARC camps I had seen on television, guerrillas told me that they had built them with permanence in mind, using different, more durable materials. While most of the houses were on the upper side of the ZVNT, my *caleta* ("sleeping area," in FARC jargon) was in the lower area. It was one among roughly twenty other huts and *caletas* that belonged to the midrank commanders and guerrillas designated to be the protective guards of 'Mauricio Jaramillo,' the FARC's Eastern Bloc commander and leader of the Colinas ZVNT.

Despite a night of insufficient rest, I started that morning full of energy and curiosity. I got my little backpack ready, came out of the mosquito net, and left the *caleta* I had been assigned. I walked toward the house of 'Mauricio Jaramillo,' whom I had met the day before. After seeing him on the news many times, mostly because he participated in the peace dialogues in Havana, it was very strange to be standing in front of him, shaking his hand, and talking to him. Peace allows unlikely, never-imagined things to happen, I thought.

On my way, I found Francisco, the midranking commander who had facilitated my access to the Colinas disarmament camp. He asked Carlos, another guerrilla member, to accompany me to the *rancha* ("cooking area," in FARC slang) to have breakfast. Still protected by the shadow of the trees, Carlos and I took a short walk, crossed a stream on a huge tree trunk, and passed

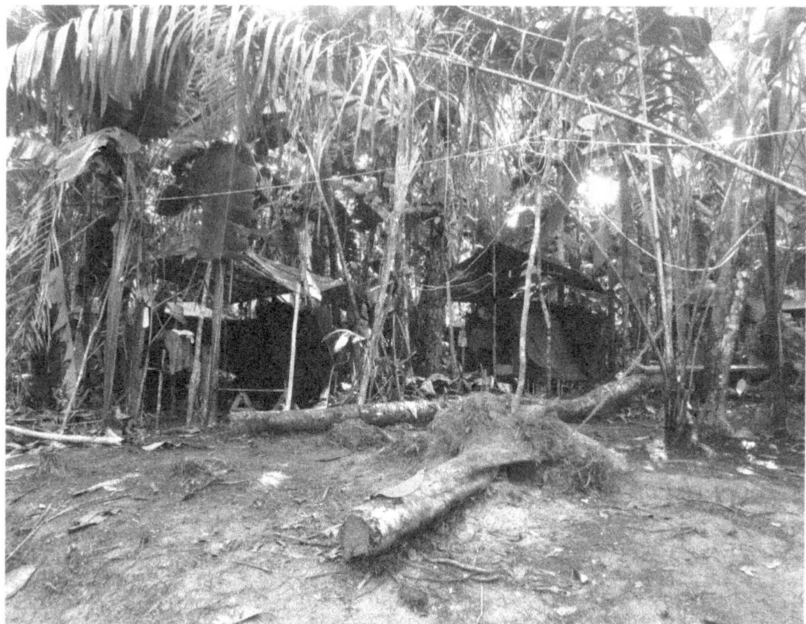

FIGURE 2.1. Makeshift huts built by FARC (ex-)guerrillas in the Colinas ZVNT. Photo by Lina Pinto-García.

by makeshift storehouses where piles of mattresses and tons of nonperishable food were being kept (fig. 2.2). Where the mass of trees ended—right on the forest's edge—a female guerrilla served me an abundant plate of noodle soup, an *arepa*, and a cup of chocolate. From there, we could see civilians and guerrillas working under the burning sun on the construction of the town.

Carlos's marked *paisa* accent—characteristic of a region in northwestern Colombia—was undeniable proof that he had grown up in Antioquia. He told me he had joined the FARC nineteen years ago when he was still a minor. He asked about the purpose of my visit. After explaining it to him, we had a conversation about leishmaniasis. During all those years, he had been infected with the disease about three times, maybe more—he could not remember. All his leishmaniasis skin lesions had been treated with Glucantime ampoules that were injected into his buttocks. He recalled that each of those treatments involved very unpleasant sensations such as chills, headaches, weakness, dizziness, and vomiting. But his last Glucantime treatment was the toughest. The drug's toxicity made him so sick that he had to divide the daily dose into smaller ones, injected throughout the day, which helped him feel a little better. I asked Carlos how the FARC had managed to maintain relatively consistent access to the treatment during the war. "There's always someone selling it. Sellers come by from time to time offering Glucantime. It's always a different seller, and I don't know exactly where they get it from. We don't ask them, and the sellers won't tell us either because that's how they make money."

As I previously discussed, the leishmaniasis public health strategy in Colombia has been completely pharmaceuticalized and centered on Glucantime.

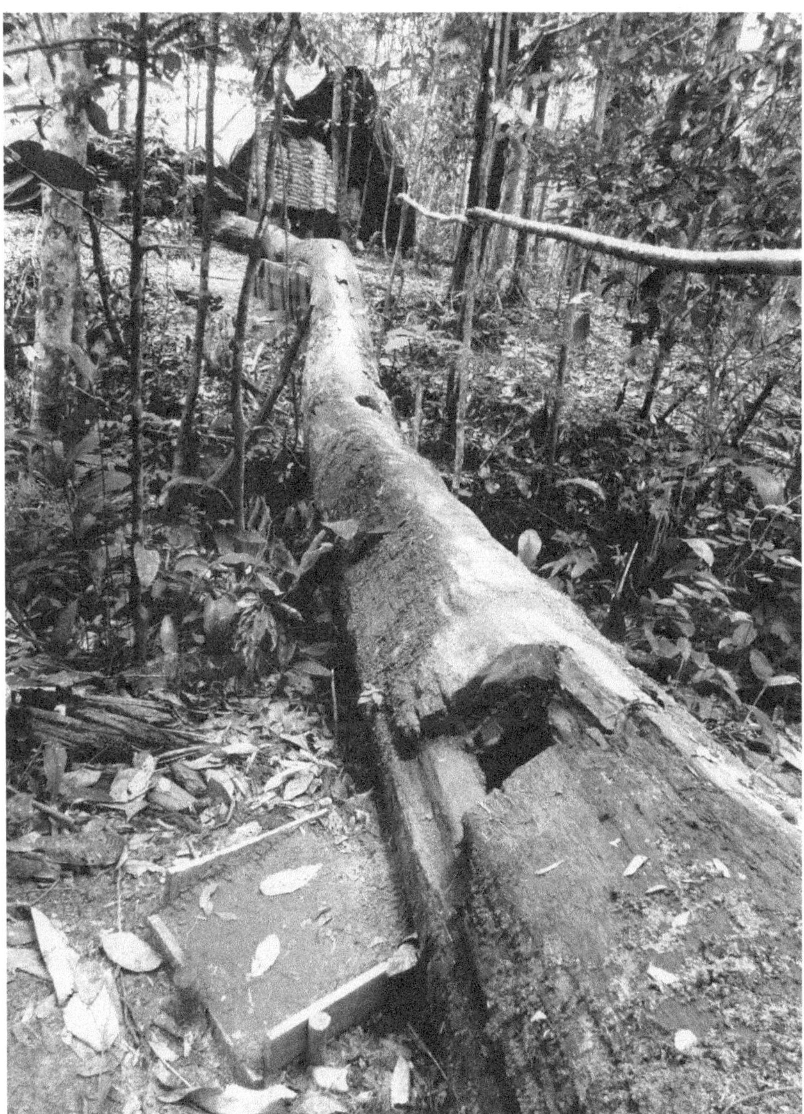

FIGURE 2.2. Infrastructures made by FARC (ex-)combatants in the Transitional Zone for Normalization (ZVNT) in Colinas, Guaviare. Photo by Lina Pinto-García.

Thus, this is the antileishmanial drug that typically circulates in the country. All legal ampoules of this medicine are purchased and imported by the Ministry of Health (MinSalud). Then, through a highly bureaucratized and drawn-out process, MinSalud distributes the drug via state health institutions to clinics and hospitals that provide health care services. In the case of the Army, the Police, the Navy, and the Air Force, collectively known in Colombia as the Public Force, the ampoules move directly from MinSalud to the *direcciones de sanidad* (health offices) of each of these institutions. Each health office then autonomously decides how to deliver the drug to its respective members affected by the disease. However, Glucantime also moves along an underground circuit that works through various clandestine mechanisms to meet the demands of guerrillas, paramilitary organizations, and people in rural Colombia who have been unable to access the treatment through legal means. This access route to Glucantime enabled people like Carlos to get treatment throughout the many years of war.

In this chapter, I trace the different circuits through which Glucantime moves in conflict-ridden Colombia. I follow this drug's trajectories from the moment it crosses into national territory until it reaches the populations of soldiers, guerrillas, and civilians affected by leishmaniasis. Glucantime has been designed to move along the legal paths established by health authorities based on scientific, material, and discursive reasonings, which I explore in detail. I also delve into the surreptitious, *extralegal* routes through which the drug circulates in conflict zones. Drawing on Carolyn Nordstrom (2009) and Alan Smart and Filippo M. Zerilli (2014), I refrain from using the term *illegal* to talk about the Glucantime routes that fall outside of legitimacy. I prefer the broader term *extralegal*, which "avoids a dichotomy between legal and illegal, encourag[ing] attention to fuzzy or contested boundaries between these domains" (Smart and Zerilli 2014, 222). Given the participation of the military and state officials in the Glucantime black market, *extralegality* is useful to examine "activities beyond the strictly legal carried out by rulers as well as the more common focus on the illegalities of the ruled" (Smart and Zerilli 2014, 222).

I show that the Glucantime ampoules entering and circulating legally in Colombia are distributed through a complex control scheme that serves to manage populations and produce therapeutic distinctions between state allies (members of the Army) and state enemies (guerrillas and civilians with uncertain affiliations). Alex Nading's work is useful here to help us think of Glucantime as a *leaky thing*—a pharmaceutical with the capacity to "drift from spaces of biomedical control and bureaucratic surveillance to ones of situated social and political interaction" (2017, 142), developed and sustained by the war in Colombia. I argue that the restrictions applied to the circulation of and access to Glucantime have turned this medicine into a biopolitical instrument of war, capable of reproducing and reinforcing a social order generated by the armed conflict. Following wartime rationales, the circulation of legal Glucantime determines which subjects are included (state allies) and which are excluded (state enemies). Thus, any person who seeks institutionalized medical attention to alleviate their leishmaniasis symptoms faces a pharmaceutical regime that simultaneously acts as a biopolitical war regime, dividing people into friends and foes. Consequently, this drug is a crucial element in the *maraña* formed by leishmaniasis and the conflict. It is through Glucantime that the governance of leishmaniasis and the social order established by armed violence come together and mutually constitute each other in a process I call the *pharmaceuticalization of war*.

Glucantime: A Core Element of the *Maraña*

While I was in Colinas in early 2017, there were six suspected cases of leishmaniasis among the nearly five hundred guerrilla members in the disarmament camp. Although smear samples had been collected a month before by health care practitioners working for the public hospital in San José del Guaviare, these six *guerrilleros* and *guerrilleras* had not yet received the diagnostic test results. Without a parasitological confirmation of leishmaniasis—the observation of parasites under the microscope—the hospital could not send Glucantime to these patients.

There were only two tattered and dusty boxes of Glucantime, one containing five ampoules and the other three, at the FARC infirmary in Colinas (fig. 2.3). Both boxes came from Venezuela, were manufactured in January 2013 in Brazil, and would expire within a year of my visit (fig. 2.4). According to the clinical protocol recommended by MinSalud, these eight ampoules were insufficient to treat even one of the six suspected cases of leishmaniasis in Colinas.[2] Although the implementation of the peace agreement between the government and the FARC had initiated three months before, the providers of these Glucantime vials were not state health institutions, as perhaps might be expected. On the contrary—these ampoules were remnants of the same black market that had met the FARC's demand for this drug throughout years of war. The lack of state-supplied Glucantime in Colinas was yet another indicator of insufficient commitment and efficiency on the part of state institutions to provide the necessary conditions for guerrilla (ex-)combatants to start making the transition to peace.

Alexandra Molina was one of the guerrilla nurses in Colinas. Although she was born in a town in Meta,[3] Alexandra and her mother moved to Bogotá

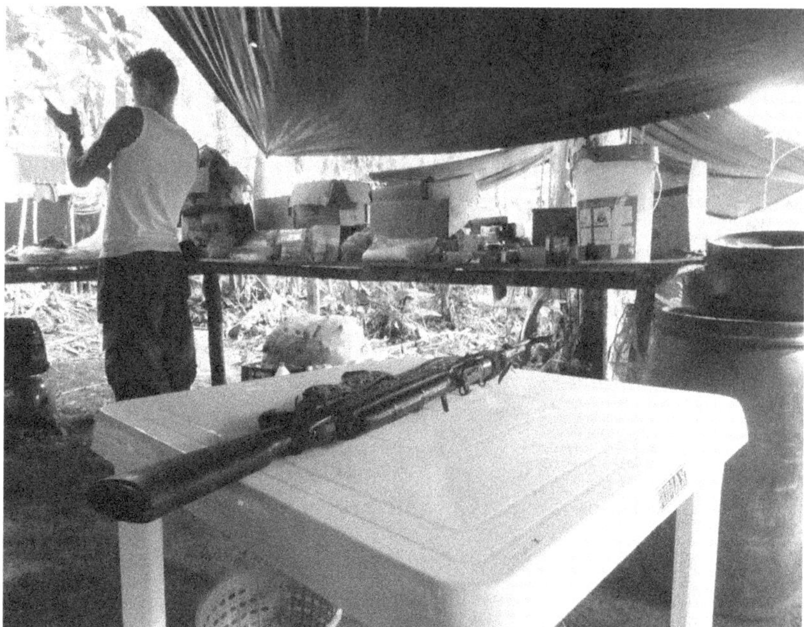

FIGURE 2.3. FARC infirmary in the Colinas ZVNT. Photo by Lina Pinto-García.

when she was a few months old, in search of better life opportunities for both of them. Once she graduated from high school, she enrolled in a university to study bacteriology. Soon after, however, her mother lost her job and Alexandra could not afford to pay for her second semester. This, she said, was one of the reasons why she went back to Meta and joined the FARC in the late 1990s. Because of her interest in health issues, she was offered the chance to work as a guerrilla nurse for the organization, a responsibility she very much enjoyed. When we spoke, she was hoping her substantial experience would be at least partially recognized in a formal capacity so that she could find a similar job *en la civil* (in civilian life). I was intrigued by the question of the accessibility of Glucantime, and she shared with me her thoughts on why it was so difficult to obtain it:

> Because the armed struggle exists. It was simply to force us to suffer the needs and consequences of the disease. The state did it more as a method of war than as a method of control. It was a strategy of war. Anyone can see that, *mi reina*. Look, when the Army came here [to the jungle], they left infected with the disease. Then, they imagined that we [guerrillas] were much worse off, we who never left the jungle. They imagined that the health problem we had with leishmaniasis was a truly complex one, so they thought that restricting and hogging all the medication would make us get out of the jungle. The military

> thought we were going to become exasperated and feel the urgent necessity to get out and expose ourselves. And, in that way, it would have been much easier for them to arrest us.

Alexandra's words show how the limited access to antileishmanial drugs in conflict zones is just one example of a classic counterinsurgency warfare strategy, often referred to as *draining the water* or *draining the swamp*, which reverses Mao Zedong's guerrilla tactic of moving through the population like fish in water. By removing civilian support ("the water") from the guerrilla movement, the exasperated insurgents ("the fish") would be exposed.[4] In this case, by restricting the circulation of pharmaceutical products from the civilian sphere, guerrillas affected by leishmaniasis would be forced to expose themselves. According to Alexandra, when she became a FARC member in the late 1990s and during the 2000s,

> many of our people who went out [of the jungle] for treatment were apprehended. And not only because of leishmaniasis, but also because of different health problems such as cancer, heart problems, or other skin issues. When we couldn't solve a particular health situation here, sick guerrillas would go out and get caught. During the so-called "democratic security" [referring to the Defense and Democratic Security Policy (PSD) during Álvaro Uribe's government], there were many *enlaces* [military liaison personnel], and they used to investigate who each person visiting a hospital was. So, the FARC decided it was better not to let anyone out, and instead, we tried to meet all health needs ourselves. That's precisely why. Because of the fear that our people would be

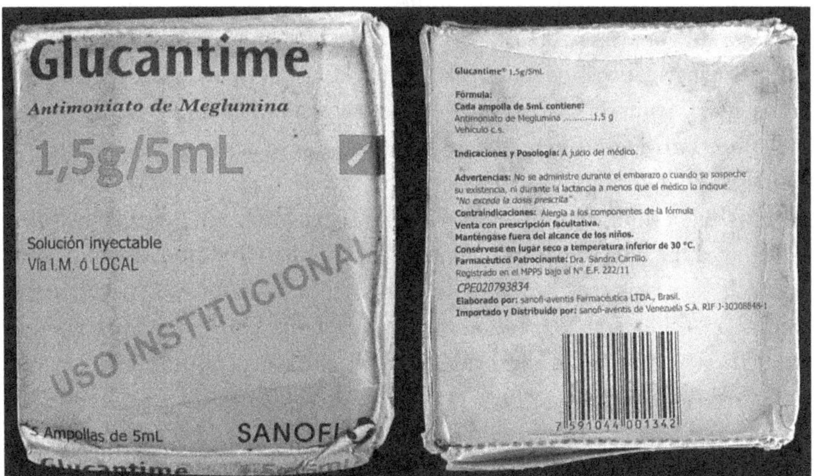

FIGURE 2.4. Front and back surfaces of one of the Glucantime boxes at the FARC infirmary in Colinas in February 2017. Photo by Lina Pinto-García.

> imprisoned. And getting imprisoned is one thing, but people who were caught were abused in many ways. Whatever the case might be, we are human beings; we are not animals.

Alexandra wasn't the only one who saw the Glucantime situation in this way. In a conversation with guerrilla commanders soon after I arrived in Colinas, these men defined Glucantime as the link connecting the disease with the war. They were referring specifically to the state's restrictive control over the drug, which they described—echoing late peace commissioner Alfredo Molano Bravo (2005b)—as a perverse antisubversive strategy. Francisco, the FARC midrank commander I met in Havana and encountered again in Colinas, said: "[Leishmaniasis] itself has no relation to the armed conflict. Its relationship with the armed conflict is the medicine to cure a tropical disease that affects the military, peasants, guerrillas, all the inhabitants of the Colombian rurality. The involvement of leishmaniasis with the armed conflict is fictitious. It's the medicine [Glucantime], the way in which the disease is treated that, in an irregular conflict like ours, like all irregular conflicts, is full of traps, trickeries, feints." Francisco identified Glucantime as the crucial link holding the *maraña* of leishmaniasis and war together. For him and the other FARC members I spoke with, there was only one way to interpret the restrictive control and access barriers applied to Glucantime: it has been a war strategy employed by the Colombian state to affect guerrilla organizations.

People in Colombia with some knowledge of leishmaniasis might know how difficult it is to access Glucantime and tend to interpret that restriction as a war practice associated with the stigma of the guerrilla disease, aimed at pressuring insurgent groups out of their dens (see, for instance, Acevedo Serna 2012). Some kidnapping survivors, for example, agree with this interpretation. Luis Eladio Pérez is a Colombian politician who was kidnapped by the FARC between 2001 and 2008 and suffered from leishmaniasis twice during this period. In an interview I conducted with him, he explained that he believed the limited access to Glucantime resulted from the idea that leishmaniasis "is a characteristic disease of guerrillas." In his view, the restrictive control over the drug "was like another weapon the state had against guerrillas; that's why they [state authorities] limited the sale of Glucantime."

It is fairly common to hear people say that Glucantime is a controlled drug in the sense that everything related to its dispensation and circulation is monitored by intelligence work undertaken by the military. I repeatedly heard that this practice allowed the Army to speculate as to who might be a guerrilla member and, according to their stigmatizing logic, target anybody looking for Glucantime. One of the many people from whom I heard this narrative was Clara Patiño, a professor at a public university who studied medicine, earned a doctoral degree in tropical medicine, and has researched leishmaniasis and other parasitic diseases in different areas of Colombia for more than three decades. She confirmed that the military had carried out intelligence work concerning Glucantime delivery in some areas of the country: "We know that this was done in the center of the country, I don't know if they continue doing it, but they did it. They did it in Cundinamarca. The doctors and staff of the San Juan de Rioseco [a municipality in eastern Cundinamarca] health service had to inform the local garrison [of the Army] who had been given Glucantime. So, there are areas of the country where we know that, indeed, the Army controlled the delivery of medicine. But this doesn't happen everywhere." Significantly, Army members have sporadically confirmed that these war reasonings have operated behind Glucantime's controlled circulation. For instance, in an article published by *El Colombiano* newspaper titled "Glucantime, the Other Dispute of the War" (Guarnizo Alvarez 2010), military dermatologist Claudia Marcela Cruz Carranza admits that the control over the drug is related to the needs of the guerrillas. Also, in a short documentary produced by TeleAntioquia in 2012 titled *Leishmaniasis, ¿Una Marca de la Guerra?* [Leishmaniasis, A Mark of War?], the then-chief of health operations of the Army, Major Omar Arturo Cabrera, said the following:

> Why is the medication controlled? In the past, the drug's price was high and the need in other areas and by other kind of people was immense, so people used to trade the drug illegally. [This happened] because the NTOs [narcoterrorist organizations, i.e., guerrillas] that are out there, many times they don't go out [from the jungle] to ask for the medicine because they don't want to expose themselves, they don't want to be seen by the Health Secretariat, the Police, or the Army. Since they [guerrillas] don't have easy access to health, what do they do? They need someone to get the medicine for them in any possible way (Acevedo Serna 2012).

As Major Cabrera describes, the restricted access to Glucantime is a strategy that has been used to antagonize guerrilla members and force them out of their hideouts. Moreover, these tactics of access control have been used to diminish their health more broadly and single out individuals as suspected guerrillas. However, to reiterate, guerrillas are not the only people in rural Colombia with leishmaniasis ulcers. Thus, the state's war strategy affects many people whose daily lives are linked in one way or another with the jungle because they either live or work in or near this forested environment.

During my time in Colinas, besides the six suspected cases I mentioned previously, there was another person affected by the disease. Javier was not a guerrilla but a civilian—a young peasant who approached his guerrilla cousin to ask for help in getting Glucantime. Appealing to my presumed expertise from having seen hundreds of leishmaniasis lesions during my fieldwork, one of the FARC commanders asked me if I could take a look at this young man's ulcer. Javier took off his hat with some shame. He gently grabbed his left ear with his fingertips and moved it a little bit forward. The lesion was huge, very infected, and about to perforate his cartilage. Worried that Javier might lose his ear, I told the FARC commanders that the young man needed antileishmanial medicine as soon as possible. Javier told us he had been diagnosed as positive for leishmaniasis several weeks ago in downtown San José, the main urban center in the *departamento* of Guaviare. In Colombia, a common excuse for the Glucantime shortage is that public health care facilities are located in rural, remote, or dispersed areas. This was not true of San José, however. Nevertheless, Glucantime was not available in the public hospital of this municipality, and Javier had not received the treatment he so urgently needed.

Javier's case is not an isolated one. People in many rural areas of Colombia confront many obstacles in accessing both diagnosis and treatment for leishmaniasis, even after the signing of the peace agreement between the state and the FARC. Approaching guerrilla organizations to obtain Glucantime ampoules is a desperate action many civilians in rural Colombia are forced to take. This became rather normal in the war context because, as I explain shortly, if anyone had leishmaniasis medicine in this country, it was either the Army or the guerrillas. Now and then, civilians would approach the FARC asking for the drug. Since people knew this armed organization regularly had Glucantime stocks, it became common for civilians to look for help from the FARC. At breakfast my first morning at the Colinas disarmament camp, Carlos told me that giving Glucantime to civilians is one of the solidarity gestures the FARC would express toward peasants—an act, among others, that allowed them to build collaborative and reciprocal relationships with the local rural population. "Peasants are very grateful and always likely to repay favors such as giving them Glucantime ampoules. Then, when you see them again, the peasant tells you 'take that bunch of bananas with you,' or 'why don't you come in and have lunch?' The downside is that assisting or collaborating with guerrillas is a crime that puts people in jail." The use of Glucantime by guerrilla organizations to create, maintain, or manipulate connections with civilians in rural Colombia is a reflection of the complicated relationships and exchanges between civilians and armed actors in these areas. In that context, lines dividing friends from foes are blurry, especially because combatants and civilians have often shared a sense of belonging to a particular territory or a long and intertwined history of friendship, solidarity, or kinship. While hatred, resentment, and fear have also marked such bonds, these are not the only kind of affective links between civilian populations to armed actors (Arjona 2016; Idler 2019). Importantly, Glucantime's role in shaping relationships between civilians and guerrillas would not be possible if obtaining the treatment through state health institutions were a simple and straightforward process, without access barriers. Actually, this particular way of weaponizing Glucantime lays bare the cumbersome and obstructive system that civilians encounter every time they approach health care institutions that are supposed to provide a free leishmaniasis diagnosis and treatment in a timely and efficient manner.

In her article "Situational Awareness," Lucy Suchman shows how the practice of differentiating "enemies" from "friends" in military operations in the Middle East has become increasingly problematic, resulting in a continuous expansion of the hostile terrain of attacks that amplifies the networks of those injured through forms of "violence at a distance" (2015, 6). Drawing on Joseph Masco's *Nuclear Borderlands* (2006), Suchman argues that technologically mediated violence has become crucial to achieving this "ever-expanding apparatus of networked warfare" (2015, 8). Although Suchman grounds her analysis in remotely operated warfare machines such as drones, I see medications like Glucantime as yet another set of technologies that becomes useful to exerting violence at a distance. In a guerrilla warfare scenario such as the one in Colombia where the political enemy is not a foreign group but armed forces made up of local people, discriminating between friends and enemies is not only challenging but is one of its most characteristic features (Wickham-Crowley 1992). While "boundaries of the battlefield are no longer clearly designated, and the sympathies of others are complex and difficult to discern" (Suchman 2015, 12), limiting access to Glucantime has been used as a war strategy to harm enemies who are likely in need of this drug. This highly unethical strategy, however, affects not only guerrilla members but also civilians in rural areas of Colombia who are not directly involved in the conflict but do coexist with it.

War is not only a matter of weapons, deaths, and injuries. War is not only an organized collection of the cruelest expressions of direct violence. War is also the manifold of forms in which biopolitical warfare emerge to control bodies in a reticular and dispersed way. The exclusionary paths through which Glucantime moves in the Colombian territory, affecting both guerrilla members and civilians, are an explicit instantiation of this.

The Bureaucratic Barriers to Glucantime Access

As I mentioned previously, MinSalud is the institution in charge of purchasing all legal ampoules of Glucantime available in Colombia. Before 2010, this ministry bought antileishmanial drugs through tender offers. Since 2010, MinSalud acquires Glucantime vials through the participation of the Colombian state in the Pan American Health Organization's (PAHO) Strategic Fund, created in September 2000. Currently, thirty-four countries and territories are members of the Strategic Fund through cooperation agreements, including many Central American and Caribbean countries and all South American countries except for French Guiana (PAHO 2023a). The list of medications that can be purchased through the Strategic Fund "utilizes the World Health Organization (WHO) Essential Medicines List (EML) as a foundation" (PAHO 2016, 7; see Greene 2011). It includes hundreds of drugs used for the treatment of a great variety of diseases (HIV, tuberculosis, malaria, cancer, leprosy, and neglected diseases such as leishmaniasis and Chagas, among others), as well as medical devices, equipment, and supplies such as insecticides, mosquito nets, and diagnostic reagents. Meglumine antimoniate (Glucantime) is one of the four antileishmanial drugs on the list, which also includes pharmaceuticals recommended as second- and third-line therapies for leishmaniasis in Colombia: amphotericin B, miltefosine, and pentamidine (PAHO 2023b).

Once Glucantime ampoules enter Colombia, they are placed under the custody of MinSalud. The drug is then distributed exclusively to the health secretariats of each of the thirty-seven territorial divisions,[5] called Departmental Health Secretariats (from here on referred to as DHSs), and the health offices of the Army, Police, Navy, and Air Force. However, the Glucantime ampoules received by the DHSs are not sent directly to hospitals and other health care facilities in the urban center of each of the 1,122 municipalities in the country.[6] Instead, there is a long and grueling multistep process before health care institutions can receive the drug to treat a leishmaniasis patient.

A person living in a remote rural area of Colombia who discovers a skin sore would probably first approach the nearest *puesto de salud* (health station). There, they would likely find not a doctor or nurse but a nursing assistant with basic medicinal supplies who does not necessarily have the education or credentials required by MinSalud to diagnose or treat leishmaniasis appropriately. Glucantime ampoules are never delivered to this kind of facility. Thus, the person would most likely be told to go, at their expense, to the closest public hospital or clinic in the *cabecera municipal* (the municipality's urban center). Although a relatively efficient road network connects several areas of Colombia, 68 percent of the country lacks even a basic transportation infrastructure (Narvaez 2017). Thus, traveling from a leishmaniasis-endemic area—geographically remote and dispersed—to the nearest urban center typically requires a substantial amount of money and unpaid time that many people who live in these areas cannot afford (Arteta 2018; MinSalud 2022). This situation is even more difficult for women who cannot leave their children unsupervised or with a friend or relative for several days (Vélez et al. 2001).

At the *cabecera municipal*, the health care staff would ask the patient if they had come from an endemic area and recently been in the jungle. Then, if the health care practitioner is familiar with leishmaniasis, which is rarely the case, they would visually examine the sore to determine if it looks like a leishmaniasis lesion. If it does, a smear sample would be taken with a scalpel blade and spread onto microscope slides. When *Leishmania* parasites are seen under the microscope—which requires a skilled practitioner not always available in the clinical facilities of the *cabeceras municipales*—the patient is reported to the national public health surveillance system (SIVIGILA) as a new leishmaniasis case. Next, one of the slides and the patient's leishmaniasis report form would be sent to the appropriate DHS in the *departamento*'s capital. Once the DHS staff receives the slide and confirms the diagnosis, the necessary Glucantime dose is calculated based on the patient's weight. Only after this lengthy process are the Glucantime ampoules released by the DHS and sent to the health care facility where the patient was initially diagnosed. Several days might pass between the sample retrieval and the arrival of the ampoules at the health care facility. If the patient is able to stay in the area for that period or leaves and returns once the ampoules arrive, several laboratory tests are required to ensure that they are healthy enough to withstand Glucantime's toxicity. These tests can be performed only if the patient can obtain the authorization from their health insurance company—known in Colombia as *Entidad Promotora de Salud*—which would cover the cost of these procedures. If the authorization is granted to test the patient, if the results are satisfactory, and if the patient can afford to stay in the urban center for another twenty days, only then would they receive the daily Glucantime injection under medical supervision. As a rule, no patient is ever given the ampoules to take home.

The number of Glucantime ampoules purchased by MinSalud corresponds to the number of leishmaniasis cases reported to the state in the previous years as well as to the more recent weekly reports that ostensibly reflect the up-to-date epidemiological behavior and spatial distribution of the disease. Even though MinSalud buys enough Glucantime to meet the national demand—based on the cases reported to SIVIGILA—the bureaucratic and geographic distance that separates most rural leishmaniasis patients from Glucantime is experienced as a huge barrier to accessing treatment. The many obstacles to obtaining Glucantime in Colombia contravene the primary aim of the PAHO Strategic Fund, whose purpose is to enable member states to obtain low-priced and high-quality drugs that are promptly and continuously delivered to the populations in need (PAHO 2018).

Glucantime Is a Controlled Medication

Why is it so difficult to be legally treated with Glucantime in Colombia? Why must it be so challenging to access this pharmaceutical even in places where leishmaniasis occurs in large numbers, year after year? *El Glucantime es un medicamento controlado* (Glucantime is a controlled medication). This is the reply I regularly received when I queried Army members, physicians, nurses, civilian patients, kidnapping survivors, guerrillas, and scientists about the challenges of obtaining Glucantime. It is a well-known fact that this drug is difficult to obtain from hospitals and clinics, let alone in rural areas where only precarious *puestos de salud* (health stations) might be available. Some of these people stated that the only way to acquire this drug is through the Army. Many found it strange that Glucantime is not available at pharmacies, as almost any other type of drug can be purchased at pharmacies without a medical prescription. In fact, it is standard practice to go to a pharmacy for medications before consulting a doctor. In urban areas, it is also common to ask a pharmacy to deliver a wide variety of pharmaceuticals with no prescription. Similarly, injections are often administered at pharmacies with no medical prescription (Vacca et al. 2005).[7]

Alicia Valencia has more than thirty years' experience in the area of public health working for the public sector. For the last ten years, she worked on a MinSalud team in charge of the national programs for surveillance and control of vector-borne diseases. This team is responsible for developing, evaluating, and updating policies related to the management of these diseases at the national level. Another of their duties is buying antileishmanial drugs through the PAHO Strategic Fund and sending them to the DHSs and health offices of the Public Force. "Why is it that people often say that Glucantime is a controlled medication?" I asked Alicia. For her, this was a misleading description of Glucantime's status in Colombia because it implied that the state or Army were restricting access to the drug as a way to harm guerrillas. In her view, the procedures established for the health care of leishmaniasis patients were designed through a universalist approach, capable of assisting all Colombians in an impartial, apolitical, and nondiscriminatory manner. She claimed that the existing system works regardless of the patient's affiliation with a guerrilla or paramilitary group. Thus, according to Alicia, this idea of "control" should be dismissed as a myth. "That is a myth, it is a myth. In Colombia, it is a myth and it is a myth for one simple reason: because, in Colombia, the medicines are acquired by the Ministry [of Health] and the Ministry distributes it to the regional [health] institutions [Departmental Health Secretariats], and also to the Military Forces. Civilians, including all those who belong to armed groups outside the law,[8] they all access the medicine as a civilian at any IPS [health care institution] for free. This means that the medication is not controlled, there is no control scheme." Alicia's words mirrored the perspective documented by anthropologist Sjaak van der Geest when WHO's Action Program on Essential Drugs was evaluated for the first time in the late 1980s. According to van der Geest, the resulting report "implicitly suggested that if the essential drug program existed on paper it existed in reality, that it was both available and used by sick people in local communities" (2006, 305). Realizing that the word *control* would not get me very far in my conversation with Alicia, I told her that I had been doing fieldwork in Candelario. This, I explained, allowed me to discover that a network of community members—the so-called *microscopists*—had been trained to diagnose malaria and dispense antimalarial drugs in rural areas, even in places far from the urban center of that municipality (Pinto-García 2023). "Why doesn't that happen in the case of leishmaniasis? What is the reason why leishmaniasis medicines don't circulate more freely, as in the case of malaria medicines?" I asked Alicia. For her, the answer to that question had three parts. First, the reason only MinSalud was allowed to buy and distribute antileishmanial drugs was based on the definition of leishmaniasis as an *event of public health interest*:

> In the world of disease surveillance and control, there are events that are of interest to the entire world population. An event of public health interest is an event that could potentially cause a pandemic. So, the interesting thing is that if we control these kinds of events, we are decreasing the risk that they will be transmitted to the entire world population. It's up to us to do surveillance and control to avoid the spreading [of these diseases]. Leishmaniasis is part of those events of public health interest. So, since it's an event of public health interest, the state has an obligation to supply the medicine, let's say, to prevent this type of disease expansion.

Alicia also told me that this "event of public health interest" terminology came from the International Health Regulations (IHR), which constitutes the legal framework that has governed infectious diseases globally since 2005. Whereas the 1969 version of the IHR was concerned with several distinct diseases (cholera, plague, and yellow fever) (Fidler and Gostin 2006; WHO 2009), the current 2005 IHR focuses on "the much more broadly conceived notion of *events* that may constitute a public health emergency of international concern" (French and Mykhalovskiy 2013, 178, emphasis in the original).[9] According to Alicia, leishmaniasis was just one among many diseases and health conditions considered to be events of public health interest in Colombia. "So are tuberculosis, leprosy, malaria, all those communicable diseases for which notification to the national public health surveillance system is mandatory," she said (see also MinSalud 1998; INS 2019). Thus, for various diseases and medical conditions so defined, MinSalud assumes the responsibility for purchasing and distributing the drugs.

She also told me that leishmaniasis and tuberculosis (TB) were comparable in terms of the risks associated with the toxicity of the pharmaceuticals and the necessity to ensure treatment adherence to avoid the emergence of drug resistance. Thus, in Alicia's view, the second reason for Glucantime's restricted circulation was that the drug was highly toxic. This fact forced health authorities to take strict precautions regarding the distribution and administration of Glucantime and of TB drugs. These same precautions are not necessary in the case of malaria, she said, because the medicine to treat it is taken orally and is nontoxic. "For these cases [leishmaniasis and TB], we [MinSalud] provide the medications, but the idea is to supervise the treatment strictly. This need for supervision forces the medications to be delivered only to those institutions able to guarantee that the patient will adhere to the treatment and that the treatment will be followed up." Thus, for Alicia, the ways that legal Glucantime ampoules are circulated are not that different from those of similarly toxic drugs employed for other "events of public health interest" such as TB. In these two cases, she considered it necessary to monitor the movement and administration of the medications to ensure their safe and responsible use, under strict conditions of medical supervision and treatment adherence. These conditions, she said, unfortunately could not be guaranteed in all clinical facilities, which, for her, also explained why the drugs were not available everywhere.

Interestingly, an anthropologist, a public health official, and a biomedical scientist working on TB confirmed to me that TB drugs are also exclusively purchased by MinSalud. However, MinSalud continuously delivers these medicines via DHS and Municipal Health Secretariats to clinics and hospitals, which means that these facilities have permanent stocks of TB medicines. The three researchers also agreed that, in the case of TB, this type of state control has led to better treatment access, adherence, and supervision. In Valle del Cauca (a *departamento* in southwestern Colombia), for example, the DHS and the Municipal Health Secretariats collaborate with health care facilities so that TB patients have consistent access to TB medications. In the city of Medellín, shortages rarely occur, and various clinics work with a network of *pares comunitarios* (community peers) who bring the medicine to patients on motorcycles and supervise the treatment.

The situation for leishmaniasis is radically different. As I have mentioned, hospitals and clinics never have Glucantime in stock.[10] Moreover, the restrictive state control over this drug has not translated into better access to treatment but rather the opposite. The therapeutic itinerary explained previously for a patient to follow in order to be diagnosed and treated is a major ordeal, full of pitfalls and contingencies that can easily go wrong—and frequently do. In addition, there is no community support in rural areas to improve health care access or treatment adherence.

During our discussion, Alicia brought up a third reason for the limited access to Glucantime: the danger of unauthorized groups stealing or seizing the drug by force. For her and the other MinSalud public officers I interviewed, this risk, which stems from guerrillas' and other armed actors' need for anti-leishmanial treatments, plays an important role in explaining the unavailability of the drug:

> The Ministry of Health acquires the medicine and delivers it to the Departmental Health Secretariats. Although we have been telling Departmental Health Secretariats to *desconcentrar* [decentralize] the drug to the health provider network [health care facilities] since 2013, they are not doing it. Instead, they keep distributing it according to the demand. Why do they do that? Because of the armed conflict. The provider network does not accept to have a stock [of Glucantime] because this drug is usually stolen. Armed groups show up and steal it or threaten them [health care workers] to get the medicine. So, in order to avoid these problems, they prefer the medication to be kept by the Departmental Health Secretariats and, according to the demand, they [health care workers] request them [the specific number of ampoules needed from the DHS]. But that is a gigantic barrier for the population to have access to the drug.

Thus, Alicia believes that another explanation for Glucantime's inaccessibility is related to "security conditions, not in relation to the *seguridad* [safety[11]] of the drug as such, but the security of the drug as a public good that can be stolen." Since this drug is considered a public good desired by enemies of the state, it becomes necessary to protect it and keep it as far away from their criminal hands as possible.

The story of Marcela Parra highlights the third point Alicia made regarding Glucantime's availability. A bacteriologist, she has led the vector-borne disease division in a DHS for more than fifteen years. While leishmaniasis is common in Marcela's geographic area of influence, she told me that her work is mainly focused on malaria—a disease that takes priority over leishmaniasis because it is more prevalent and potentially fatal. While malaria treatments circulate and are always available in the areas Marcela is responsible for, even in remote and dispersed rural zones, Glucantime ampoules are carefully stockpiled in the building where she works. According to Marcela, this restriction on Glucantime ampoules was established because "guerrillas used to steal the medicine." She told me that, in the early 2000s, this had happened at the hospital of one of the largest municipalities under her territoral jurisdiction. "They [guerrillas] came to the hospital pharmacy and took all the medication," she said. For that reason, Marcela and her colleagues decided that they would concentrate all Glucantime in the DHS facility and dispense the exact number of ampoules required for each patient only after receiving a microscope slide showing that parasites were visible. That measure, however, was not entirely effective.

> Still, and I'm going to be honest with you, there was more than one attempt [of armed actors] to demand the medication here [at that particular DHS]. However, I never consented to do that. I always asked them to please not do that. I told them this: "I don't care if you tell me your real name or not, or if you make up your ID number. I'm only interested in having your smear taken, confirming that you're positive, measuring your weight and, if you can, have your lab tests results. Otherwise, I can't give you that medication, please be understanding."

In this way, Marcela persuaded armed actors to refrain from taking the medication by force on several occasions. One of her colleagues, however, a recent hire with no experience handling such matters, did hand over Glucantime ampoules to guerrillas. "She told me she had been pressured," Marcela said with regret. After that, Marcela handled these unwanted visits personally. As a result, they decreased with time.

Returning to Alicia's three explanations for the limited access to Glucantime, each rationale is based on different arguments. First is a regulatory argument, stemming from terminology and mandates from multilateral health organizations that the Colombian state must follow to avoid the international spread of the disease. For health authorities, the definition of leishmaniasis as an *event of public health interest* explains why MinSalud is the only entity authorized to buy all available Glucantime ampoules and distribute them via state health institutions—as is the case for malaria, TB, leprosy, and other infectious health conditions. Second, a medico-scientific argument emphasizes Glucantime's toxicity as the reason why it would be irresponsible for the state not to treat leishmaniasis patients under medically supervised and clinically contained conditions—as is the case for TB. Because these two arguments are not exclusive to leishmaniasis, they do not provide much insight into the specifics of Glucantime's limited availability. Furthermore, when looking at how treatment access differs for leishmaniasis, TB, and malaria, it is evident that neither argument can fully explain why leishmaniasis patients face such insurmountable barriers. Malaria and TB are also defined as events of public health interest, but the pharmaceuticals to treat these diseases are accessible. Moreover, TB therapy is as toxic as Glucantime and requires the careful supervision of medical personnel, but TB patients are still able to access the drugs.

Alicia's third argument is specific to leishmaniasis: the unavailability of Glucantime is due to security imperatives imposed by the war and needs of armed actors. According to this rationale, health care institutions responsible for diagnosing, reporting, and treating leishmaniasis patients face the challenge of supplying the medicine while also preventing guerrillas and other armed actors from obtaining it. As a result, the drug is hardly available to those in need, whether they are guerrillas, paramilitaries, or civilians. By prioritizing a war logic and imperatives over finding a solution to a public health problem, Colombian health authorities in Colombia have *not only allowed but also accepted* the establishment of various obstacles to accessing Glucantime. While public health interests and medical concerns maintain an important place in state decisions to treat leishmaniasis patients, the war is a key element in the therapeutic management of the disease in Colombia.

Although public health and war may seem to be unrelated state issues, the restrictions imposed on Glucantime show how these two factors are interconnected and result deeply *enmarañados* in the context of a long-standing and pervasive war. Contrary to the opinions of Alicia and other public health officials, I have documented that a complex Glucantime control scheme created through a variety of discourses, practices, and expertise is precisely what has been deeply entrenched throughout years of armed conflict. While the establishment of these barriers has prevented insurgents from appropriating the drug—forcing them out of the jungle and making them more vulnerable to detentions—it has also resulted in the systemic neglect of rural citizens affected by leishmaniasis. In other words, not only those labeled as enemies by the state are affected by this strict control but also everyone else whose daily lives are entangled with the forests and territories ravaged by conflict, disease, and inequality.

The pattern of Glucantime's (un)availability in Colombia is largely defined by public health concerns, medical precautions related to the drug's toxicity, and perverse war strategies of inclusion and exclusion inherited from many years of state-sanctioned violence and devastation. I call this process of mutual configuration between wartime social orders and pharmaceutical regimes the *pharmaceuticalization of war*. On the one hand, this conceptual resource is useful in highlighting the incorporation of a pharmaceutical into war practices, strategies, and logic. On the other hand, it indicates that Glucantime's control scheme does not randomly exclude people but follows a long-standing pattern that divides rural residents into state allies and state enemies (see Jimeno 2001).

It is important to reiterate that this type of social fragmentation is highly ambiguous in the context of a guerrilla warfare where civilians are not easily set apart from members of armed organizations. Thus, while guerrillas have been the main target of Glucantime's restrictions, they are not the main victims. Guerrillas, after all, have been powerful actors in rural Colombia and have managed to access the drug despite the restrictions imposed by state health authorities. As is often the case with armed conflicts, and especially Colombia's war, civilians living in the middle of war tend to be the main victims of various types of violence. Likewise, Glucantime's control scheme has mostly affected rural populations who struggle to survive among armed actors violently disputing territorial control and civilian support. The harmful effects of Glucantime's unavailability on civilians, however, should not be understood as a "collateral damage" of a sophisticated war strategy deployed through a pharmaceutical. As the CNMH report states: "For decades, the victims were ignored behind the legitimizing discourses of war, vaguely recognized under the generic label of the civilian population or, even worse, under the pejorative descriptor of 'collateral damage.' From this perspective, victims were considered a residual effect of the war and not the core of war regulations" (CNMH 2013, 14). In areas where leishmaniasis is endemic, the restricted circulation of Glucantime has reproduced a war order concerned with state enemies as well as civilians who are frequently understood as an extension of guerrillas. In war zones, paramilitary groups and the state armed forces have systematically used expressions such as *guerrillas' collaborators* or *guerrillas' social bases* to justify violence against civilians (CNMH 2013, 38). Thus, the damage caused by the pharmaceuticalization of war also incorporates these forms of logic through which violence, although indiscriminate, can always be justified by sowing doubt about the "real" affiliations of civilians in rural Colombia and the "real" motivations behind their actions. The stigma that characterizes leishmaniasis in Colombia serves this purpose well, as it opens the way for people affected by the "guerrilla disease" to be treated like guerrillas: state enemies deserving nothing but violence.

Soldiers Enjoy Privileged Access to Glucantime

Civilian access to Glucantime has been challenging, but the situation for the state armed forces has been radically different, particularly since the 2000s. According to official figures, Colombia's military population has the highest incidence of leishmaniasis and is considered "the most vulnerable group, due to the continuous deployment of troops to areas of high endemicity and high circulation of the insect vector" (Patino et al. 2017, 2). Soldiers who come out of the jungle with skin lesions receive a diagnosis and twenty days of Glucantime treatment (twenty-eight days in the case of mucosal leishmaniasis) under medical supervision. Civilians affected by leishmaniasis do not enjoy the same specialized care, medical attention, access to diagnosis and medication, or follow-up. It should be noted, though, that this unequal access to medical care is not unique to leishmaniasis. As Emily Cohen (2015) points out, a similar pattern is observed in the case of land mine victims and their access to surgical amputation and rehabilitation—while soldiers receive the best medical care available in Colombia, civilians do not (see also CNMH and Fundación Prolongar 2017).

Since soldiers constitute a population whose health status has been extremely relevant for the state's war purposes, they have been treated in a significantly different way than civilians. Although at least half of the people affected by leishmaniasis are not in the military, regarding medical care, soldiers represent a highly privileged population. This is especially evident in the unequal distribution of Glucantime between the Army and civilians. According to a MinSalud public servant, even though Army soldiers accounted for half of the leishmaniasis cases reported to SIVIGILA during the mid-2000s, "of every six [leishmaniasis] patients, five medications were [allocated to] the Army and one to the civilian population." As a result of the peace process, the number of leishmaniasis cases reported to the state has fallen by 17 percent (Iza Rodríguez, Iza Rodríguez, and Olivera 2021). According to the same source, this caused a shift in how Glucantime is distributed, and "we now have most of the drugs in the Departmental Health Secretariats and the rest is in the Army."

The imbalance in the distribution of Glucantime during the harshest years of the armed conflict had important effects on how the *enmarañamiento* of war, leishmaniasis, and this pharmaceutical have been understood and experienced. In Colombia, it is common to hear not only that the treatment for leishmaniasis is exclusively controlled by the state but also that it is specifically controlled by the Army. This perception results from widely spread stories about leishmaniasis sufferers in rural areas who were denied treatment at health care facilities only to obtain Glucantime after seeking assistance from Army personnel. While it is illegal for the Army to give Glucantime to nonmilitary people, a MinSalud officer admitted that this has occurred on several occasions. He explained: "As people knew that the [military] dispensary had the drug, then obviously the regular population [civilians] used to go to the Army officers for them to provide the medicine." Even though this is not the conventional or legal way for civilians to access Glucantime, the fact is that the military—like the guerrillas—have been (more than) occasional providers of the drug.

Although the Army—and other state armed forces—does not own or control the entire stock of Glucantime vials that enter Colombia, it has historically received much more Glucantime and other antileishmanial drugs than the civilian population, and soldiers have been granted extensive access to diagnosis and treatment since the mid-2000s. In the eyes of the civilian population and guerrilla organizations, this inequitable and unbalanced distribution of Glucantime is interpreted as state—and specifically military—control of the drug.

While the "universal" distribution of antileishmanial drugs is discursively performed as a state responsibility to its citizens, Glucantime has been remade into a biopolitical instrument of war to segregate populations and define who enjoys citizen status and who does not. In the context of war that prevails in Colombia, unequal access to this pharmaceutical has drawn a boundary dividing state allies and state enemies—a division that enables, in practice, the elimination of the universalist rhetoric of the right to health. As a result, soldiers are considered to be entitled to therapy access, while other leishmaniasis sufferers are labeled as either guerrillas or guerrilla collaborators who do not deserve to be healthy. Therefore, they are treated as illegitimate populations that can be excluded from access to treatment regardless of whether they are guerrillas or not.

Scholars of science and technology studies and medical anthropology have noted instances when biological or biomedical conditions provide the basis for people to make rights claims, develop a sense of belonging, gain political recognition, and access health care, resources, and some form of social inclusion—ultimately, to acquire a biologically oriented citizenship. Adriana Petryna (2004) and Nikolas Rose and Carlos Novas (2005) developed the concept of *biological citizenship* to describe how physical suffering is turned into a resource to obtain welfare in the context of neoliberal reforms. In particular, Vinh-Kim Nguyen (2010) explores how ART was initially accessible to people living with HIV in French West Africa in the late 1990s. He coined the term *therapeutic citizenship* to draw attention to "the way in which individuals living with HIV appropriate ART as a set of rights and responsibilities" (Nguyen et al. 2007, 34). Through their testimonials about being HIV positive, much like Western self-help and empowerment narratives, individuals not only received medication; they also used their illness narratives to gain access to other resources and become part of valuable social networks. Thus, therapeutic citizenship involves shaping oneself in certain ways and asserting a political right to belong to communities that provide access to health care and medications. But, in the context of drug scarcity, therapeutic citizenship is also about determining who would benefit from the limited supply of ARTs donated to HIV/AIDS groups. Nguyen defines *social triage* as the practices used by these HIV/AIDS groups to "separate those who would receive treatment and live from those who would not" (2010, 89). The concept of triage, he explains, "was initially developed in wartime, as a way to use scarce treatment resources most rationally; those most likely to live are prioritized to receive care, whereas those whose prognosis is poor are left to die" (Nguyen et al. 2007, 33). Similarly, in communities of people living with HIV, the scarcity of ARTs led to selecting the most charismatic individuals for treatment based on the persuasiveness of their testimonials: the more compelling the testimonies, the higher the likelihood of receiving medication. The rationale applied here was that these people were thought to be better equipped to advocate for donations of drugs and resources for the group. If their narratives enabled them to access the needed medications, "they would be able to help others more than those who remained passive" (Nguyen 2010, 99).

As I have shown, a similar "machinery for sorting people out" (Nguyen 2010, 13) is responsible for the unequal access to antileishmanial drugs in Colombia. A therapeutic citizenship defines who deserves state-provided pharmaceutical care and who does not. However, the social triage in place is not necessarily a result of the shortage of drugs and the consequent need to ration them, as is the case with ART access in West Africa. Instead, determining who is included and who is excluded is based on war calculations that redraw social fault lines deeply rooted in Colombia's history of conflict. The state benefits from soldiers' privileged access to Glucantime because a quicker recovery from leishmaniasis means they can return to combat sooner, as I discuss in the next chapter. Likewise, restricting guerrillas from accessing this drug benefits the state's war project. At stake is not the application of a utilitarian principle that sacrifices some lives to save many others, as is the case in Nguyen's analysis, but the elimination of a diffuse and elusive enemy, whatever the cost may be. The pharmaceuticalization of war in the case of Colombian leishmaniasis is a clear example of the inclusionary and exclusionary practices that underlie any definition of citizenship. The recognition of citizenship rights always starts from demarcating a boundary between those who bear the status of citizen and those who do not.

Extralegal Paths

In November 2016, Sergeant Ricardo Rodríguez picked me up in his car at 4:00 a.m. at a gas station outside Duitama in Boyacá. After a four-hour drive, we arrived at the Health Office of the Colombian Army (DISAN) in a central area of Bogotá. The closest building to the entrance was a warehouse where several boxes of medications, vaccines, and medical supplies were messily stored on ceiling-high shelves. Rodríguez gave the sergeant in charge of the warehouse documents stating that the head of the CRL, an Army major, had authorized Rodríguez "to pick up 5000 ampoules of meglumine antimoniate (Glucantime) to treat soldiers diagnosed with leishmaniasis in the Leishmaniasis Recovery Center." After showing his military ID and signing several papers, Rodríguez received six boxes and ten loose Glucantime packages with the five thousand ampoules. According to the documents Rodríguez gave the sergeant, MinSalud had paid 12,280,900 Colombian pesos (about USD 4,000), that is, 2,456.18 pesos per ampoule (about USD 0.8).[12] We drove back to Duitama with the precious cargo in the trunk.

Two days later, I accompanied Rodríguez to the warehouse where the medical supplies for both the Silva Plazas Battalion dispensary and the CRL were stored, as well as the Glucantime boxes we had picked up in Bogotá. These boxes were stacked next to a metal shelf filled with clusters of Glucantime packages carefully arranged by Rodríguez. Each cluster contained one to eight Glucantime packages, and each package contained ten ampoules. The first package of each cluster was open, and a handwritten surname could be read on each upper flap: "Leal," "Guzmán," "Navarro," "Martínez," "García," and so on. These were the fifty-three soldiers being treated for leishmaniasis in the CRL at that time. Rodríguez had assigned a Glucantime cluster to each of them, including the exact number of ampoules each soldier needed—not one more, not one less (fig. 2.5).

Rodríguez asked me to help him gather the ampoules needed to treat the fifty-three soldier-patients that day and the day after. He handed me a form and asked me to read out loud the surname of each soldier, the number of ampoules that each soldier needed per day (either three or four, depending on his weight), and the number of ampoules that should remain in that soldier's personal stock. Filling a fabric bag with the correct number of Glucantime ampoules took us more than an hour. Near the end of that process, two ampoules had broken, and Rodríguez carefully discarded them in the trash bin. Rodríguez told me he followed the same rigorous and laborious procedure every two days. In the end, he gave the soldier in charge of the warehouse some documents that Rodríguez had received from CRL's administrative staff, showing the exact number of ampoules he was removing from the main stock on that day. The soldier had Rodríguez

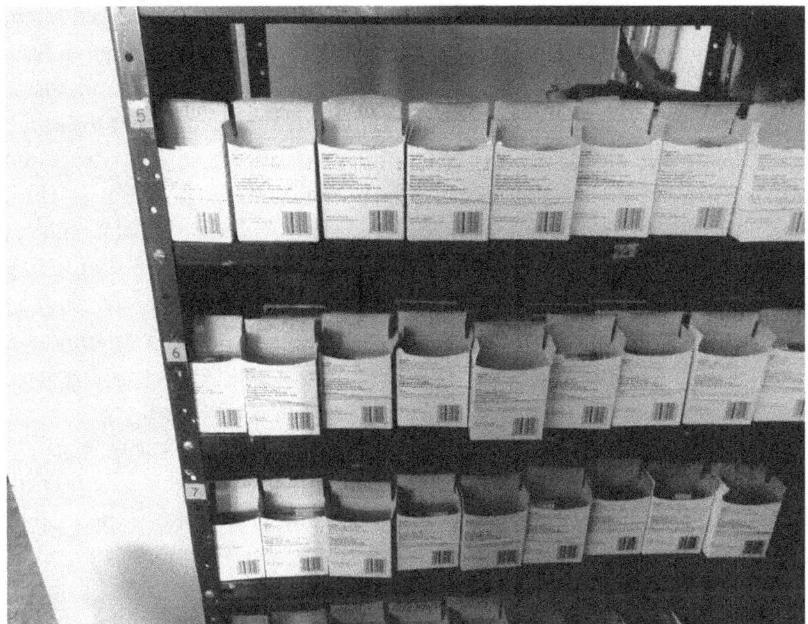

FIGURE 2.5. Personal stocks of Glucantime ampoules for each of the soldiers under treatment at the CRL. Photo by Lina Pinto-García.

sign several documents and entered the information into a computer. Finally, we carried the bag to the CRL, located several meters away.

Given the military's strict controls over the transport of Glucantime, which are supported by a rigorous accountability system that relies on meticulous recordkeeping at the DISAN, the Silva Plazas Battalion, and the CRL, I felt as if we were carrying gold or a large sum of money from one place to another. I wondered how anyone could even consider trying to divert ampoules through corrupt routes to sell them to guerrilla organizations or anyone else who traded the drug on the black market. I discussed this with several people at the CRL. While they admitted that such "unwanted losses" of ampoules from Army stocks often occurred, many said that this was why strict procedures were in place to closely monitor Glucantime's movement within the Army. When I asked if these measures actually worked, the replies were consistently ambiguous. Finally, an Army member said: "Every process has its hole, its void, and if someone wants to steal Glucantime, I assure you it can be done." "But how?" I asked incredulously, remembering how tightly the stock of each individual soldier is controlled.

Based on the patient's weight in kilograms, the daily doses of Glucantime are calculated in milliliters, not in the number of ampoules (fig. 2.6). Not all patients require exactly three (15 ml) or four (20 ml) ampoules. More often, the dose is 14.5 ml (almost three ampoules for a 59 kg patient), 16 ml (a little over three ampoules for a 65 kg patient), or 19 ml (almost four ampoules for a 77 kg patient), for example. When several men are treated one after the other, as is the case in the Army, any remaining medication can, and is required to, be used. Otherwise, this valuable drug would simply go to waste. Thus, the total number of ampoules actually administered daily to the soldiers never corresponds to the on-paper sum of ampoules—always three or four—prescribed to and injected into each soldier-patient. "At what point does the number of ampoules injected coincide with the exact number of ampoules prescribed?" I asked one of the CRL nursing assistants. "Only when we have one single patient, which is never going to happen," she replied.

A single patient requiring 16.5 ml of Glucantime daily, for example, would be treated with four ampoules (20 ml), of which 3.5 ml would be wasted. However, if there are two patients, that remaining amount would be used to complete the dose of the second patient. After treating several more patients, there will inevitably be an unopened ampoule that was not used. This leftover ampoule might be passed around through unofficial channels to fill the ongoing demand of guerrillas, paramilitaries, or civilians in rural areas. Moreover, Glucantime is stored in small glass vials—and glass can break. It is expected that when handling hundreds of ampoules to treat dozens of soldier-patients on a daily basis, as is the case at the CRL, some Glucantime vials might break—and, as I saw in the warehouse with Rodríguez, they do indeed break.

It is precisely the large number of soldiers treated at the CRL that enables the staff—physicians, nurses, and nursing and administrative assistants—to handle a broad diversity of leishmaniasis cases. Being exposed to different types of cases, the CRL staff have gained unparalleled knowledge about and experience with the disease (see chapter 3), and are thus able to provide superior care for their patients. Furthermore, the CRL's high level of control and surveillance of soldier-patients is unmatched, even at other Army medical facilities where leishmaniasis is treated. However, dealing with a large number of patients makes it impossible to predict or verify what actually happens to Glucantime used in the numerous therapeutic procedures performed in military health facilities every day. In other words, there seems to be ample room for error in Glucantime dispensation, which could lead to false claims that more ampoules were damaged or used than the actual number. These discrepancies in recordkeeping might be one way that Glucantime could escape the Army's control.

Ironically, the Army is a major source of Glucantime for the black market, which has been operating for decades during war in Colombia to meet the demand of guerrillas and other armed groups. Public servants in state health

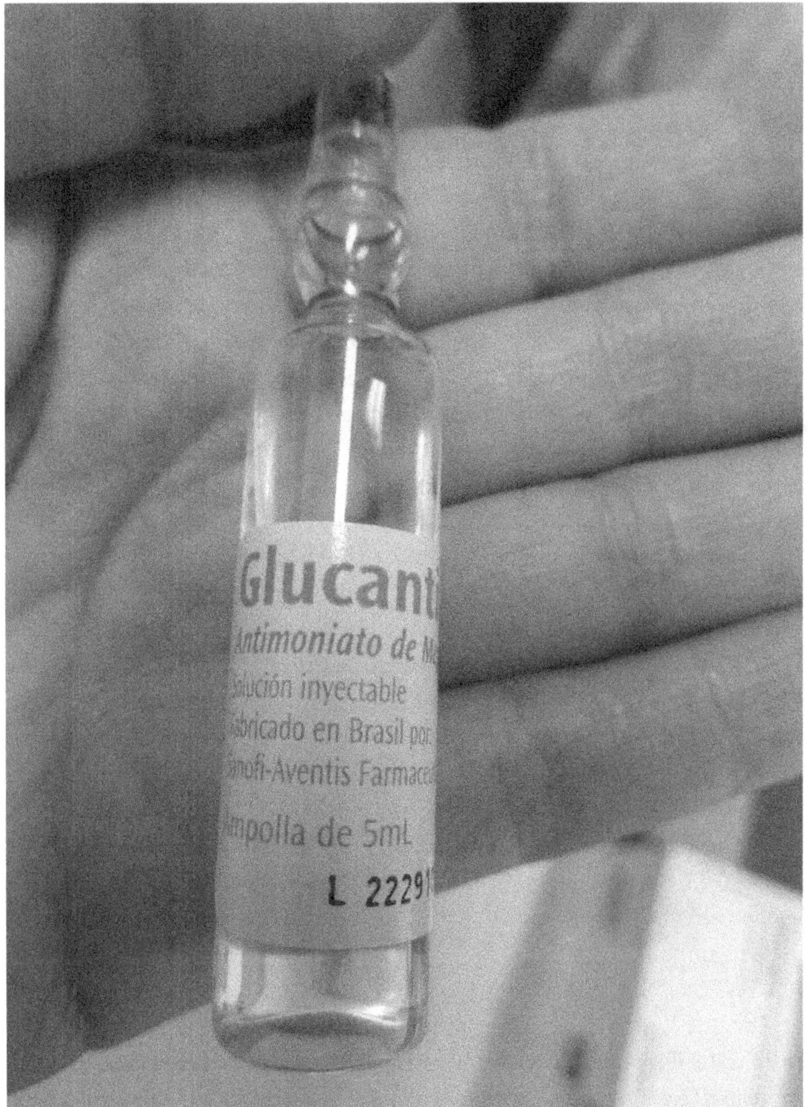

FIGURE 2.6. Glucantime ampoule. Each one contains 5 ml of the drug. Photo by Lina Pinto-García.

institutions who have direct access to the drug have also participated in these extralegal activities (see Guarnizo Alvarez 2010). Besides these corrupt networks,[13] Glucantime also enters Colombia through smugglers who somehow manage to bring in ampoules from neighboring countries[14] and find customers in the rural areas of the country.

Destabilizing the support networks of guerrilla organizations and cutting their supply lines are warfare strategies commonly employed by the Army and the Police in Colombia. Glucantime has been among the disputed goods that guerrillas try to obtain and the state armed forces try to seize. According to a 2006 cable released by WikiLeaks, leishmaniasis was known to "take a heavier toll on the FARC . . . who live full-time in jungle camps, and whose medicine supply lines are long (cross-border) and can be disrupted by COLMIL [the Colombian military] action" (US Embassy in Colombia 2006b). On several occasions, members of the Public Force confiscated hundreds of Glucantime ampoules that were found during the detainment of FARC members, when FARC members deserted, or when hideouts belonging to paramilitary or guerrilla groups were discovered.[15] Also, the media has often reported on seizures of Glucantime by the Army or Police that were allegedly intended for guerrilla groups, even in neighboring countries such as Venezuela and Brazil.[16]

In Colinas, I asked a member of the FARC Secretariat,[17] a seasoned guerrilla member with almost forty years inside the organization, how he managed to access the treatment.

"We had to buy the ampoules ourselves, it's like that," he replied.

"And who sells them?" I asked.

"Black market sellers."

"Do they come by and offer it to you, or what is it like?"

"No, it's more like selling weapons: 'Hey, brother, aren't you able to get some Glucantime?' 'Yes, yes, of course.' 'How much do you get it for?' '7, 8, 9, 10,000 pesos.' "

"And the price changes according to what?"

"According to the need and *la cara del marrano* [the person who's asking]," he said, giggling. "Some of those degenerates could charge up to 15,000 pesos."

"Per ampoule?"

"Yes."

For this FARC leader, Glucantime's black market operated on the same basis as the illegal trade of other hard-to-obtain goods that are valuable in the context of the war, like weaponry. The limited availability of Glucantime for nonmilitary populations has transformed this drug into an object of immense value. Because Glucantime is highly sought after, its price is inflated in rural areas of Colombia and also fluctuates depending on availability and the person in need. The continuing demand for this pharmaceutical leads to moneymaking opportunities. Prices have increased due to the scarce supply and the restrictions on circulating Glucantime beyond state institutions. While MinSalud used to pay 2,456.18 pesos (about USD 0.8) per ampoule in 2016, black market prices have increased from 3,000 to 4,000 pesos in the 1990s to 7,000 to 15,000 pesos in more recent years. Some FARC (ex-)combatants even mentioned prices of 27,000 pesos per ampoule, and a midrank guerrilla (ex-) commander told me that corrupt military personnel standardized the price at 12,000 pesos (see also Guarnizo Alvarez 2010).

Interestingly, in addition to being a valuable commodity traded on the black market, Glucantime has also been used as an object of deception in Colombia. For example, national news outlets have widely reported criminal groups demanding Glucantime ampoules from their victims as a means of extortion.[18] Taking advantage of Glucantime's scarcity and reputation as a substance sought after by guerrillas, criminals would demand Glucantime from their victims in order to scare them into thinking that they were being extorted by guerrilla groups. Once the victims were frightened enough by the threats of these supposed guerrillas, only to face the impossibility of obtaining Glucantime, they were more likely to comply with the criminals and give them money.

Not only unwary civilians but also guerrilla groups have fallen prey to Glucantime scams. Although corrupt military personnel typically charged 12,000 pesos for each vial, at one point, the FARC was offered a price of 10,000. Excited about the deal, FARC commanders purchased large quantities of the drug. However, when they saw how easily the ampoules reached their camps, they started to get suspicious. 'El Mono Jojoy'—a member of the FARC Secretariat and commander of the Eastern Bloc from 1990 until his assassination in 2010—realized that the ampoules did not contain Glucantime and stopped further purchasing of the drug. "It was *suero*, pure saline solution what we were getting injected," said Francisco, the FARC midrank commander who shared this story with me. Indeed, 'El Mono Jojoy' discovered that a group of soldiers had set up a factory to create fake Glucantime and were profiting from the scam. "Episodes like that have been part of the war," Francisco concluded.

A military doctor told me that the Army had discovered more fake Glucantime during a confiscation from the guerrillas. "We do not know if they [the guerrillas] wanted us to use it [fake Glucantime] seeking another result. Finally, they [the ampoules] were destroyed," she said.

The legal and extralegal circulation routes of Glucantime highlighted in this chapter define some of the components forming the *maraña* between war and leishmaniasis, where the material properties of the drug—being highly toxic, liquid, and packaged in glass vials—play a significant role. Glucantime is at the center of a biopolitical warfare strategy, implemented through a control scheme that involves public health institutions and regulations, state officials, and medical-scientific discourses. The armed conflict in Colombia has defined the pathways through which Glucantime circulates, both legally and illegally. In other words, the rules of war have significantly restricted and defined the ways in which civilians, soldiers, and armed actors can access this medication. They have determined who should be recognized as a legitimate leishmaniasis patient deserving medical treatment, and who should be stigmatized as a state enemy against whom violence is justified. The drug has colonized, leaked, and merged into the everyday reality of exclusion and violence, creating what I refer to as the pharmaceuticalization of war. Through this process, Glucantime is caught up in the *maraña*, spreading beyond its intended use as a medicine and becoming a valuable war instrument that shapes both wartime social orders and pharmaceutical practices. The patterns of inclusion and exclusion that Glucantime follows and reproduces demonstrate how pharmaceuticals can play a role in defining citizenship in a context of armed conflict. The circuits through which Glucantime moves show how war can invade every sociocultural corner of society, including spaces and actors in seemingly aseptic areas such as medicine and public health.

In Colinas, while we were contemplating a peaceful stream and some monkeys jumping from tree to tree above our heads, Francisco and I talked about what it would take to disentangle leishmaniasis and war. "It is still necessary that, as a result of the peace process, the veto against the medicine that cures leishmaniasis is lifted; it should not be restricted anymore," he said. "That is something that was not discussed in Havana," added another FARC commander who overheard our conversation. For Glucantime to no longer be used as an instrument of war, it is crucial to significantly change the bureaucracies and regulations that prevent people from accessing this medicine. This will ensure that those who need leishmaniasis therapy will receive it. But it is also important to not reduce the disentanglement of leishmaniasis and the war to a problem of accessing medications. In other words, to assume that the *enmarañamiento* of war and leishmaniasis can be fixed with a pharmaceutical solution would lead to the same conditions that caused the *maraña* in the first place. Trusting blindly in pharmaceutical technologies and their pharmaceutical regimes does not fix the problem—indeed, it might perpetuate it. It does not address or change the stigmatization of leishmaniasis sufferers. Moreover, it leaves unchallenged the systemic and historical use of a potentially deadly pharmaceutical to deal with a nondeadly disease that can, in fact, be treated in alternative ways (Pinto-García 2022). Making justice the primary objective in achieving peace means we strive not only to remove obstacles to accessing leishmaniasis medications but also to ensure that all rural communities in Colombia have full access to health care. It implies that, while embracing our ambivalent desires toward drugs and the state (Camargo and Ojeda 2017), we hold pharmaceutical regimes and health authorities accountable for the perpetuation of violence and contributing to the indefinite postponement of peace.

3
Leishmaniasis within the Colombian Army

It was 7:30 a.m. on a cold and foggy morning in the military CRL (fig. 3.1). Like any other day around that time, all soldier-patients with leishmaniasis stood in formation in the front yard. Facing them, behind a lectern, the major who led the facility made several announcements and received the morning report from the three patients with the highest military rank—three lieutenants with leishmaniasis. These officers had each been put in charge of one of the three companies (groups of about thirty men) making up the "CRL battalion" while undergoing treatment and recovery themselves. Although the CRL was not officially a battalion, as the major would explain to me later, the patients were divided into companies A, B, and C to maintain discipline and control. While the major did not need a medical background to lead the facility, training in the military sciences and substantial experience as a commander were crucial. His job, he told me, was to maintain discipline not only among soldiers undergoing leishmaniasis treatment but also the CRL staff, composed of one officer, six subofficers, and twelve civilians. In his view, discipline was particularly important when working with nonmilitary employees. If civilian personnel was left unchecked, he said, "they tended to be too *folclóricos* [behave in a relaxed manner]."

The major read aloud four lists of surnames prepared the previous afternoon by one of the CRL nurses. First came the soldiers who had to undergo laboratory tests that day either because they were about to start, were in the middle of, or had already finished their Glucantime treatment. Second in line were the soldiers who were scheduled to see one of the three general practitioners that day. Third on the list were the soldiers who had to initiate their twenty-day treatment on that day. Last were the soldiers who had shown visible signs of Glucantime intolerance and whose treatment was temporarily

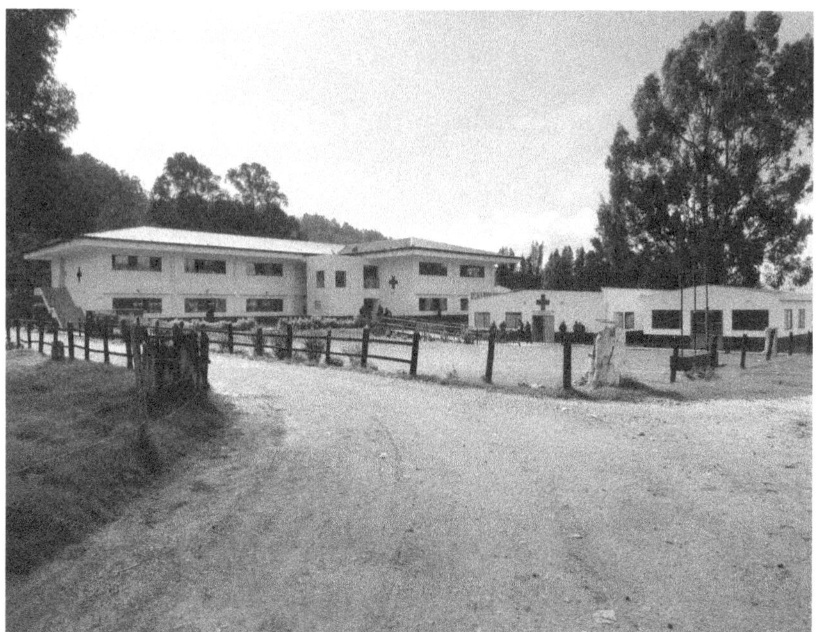

FIGURE 3.1. Leishmaniasis Recovery Center (CRL) within the Silva Plazas Battalion in Duitama, Boyacá. Photo by Lina Pinto-García.

suspended. The major then ordered those soldiers in the observation period (approximately twenty-five days after finishing the treatment) to stay in the front yard for their scarring process to be evaluated immediately by the major, the head military doctor, and one of the military nursing assistants. With no regard for privacy or the cold weather, these soldiers were told to display their leishmaniasis lesions; many had to undress partially to do so. While making harsh jokes and humiliating comments about the soldiers' appearance and their leishmaniasis ulcers, this military-medical group decided who was ready to leave the CRL and return to his respective military unit because his lesion(s) had satisfactorily healed. Meanwhile, the soldiers undergoing treatment were dispatched to the Vital Signs Room, where their weight and heart rate were measured daily and recorded on paper to monitor the weight loss and possible heart problems caused by Glucantime.

"Garcíaaaa!" Marisol's commanding voice rang out from the room next to the Vital Signs Room, calling one of the men. She was one of three nursing assistants in the Injection Room that day. García opened the door and entered. He was the first of seventy soldiers to receive two Glucantime injections that day.

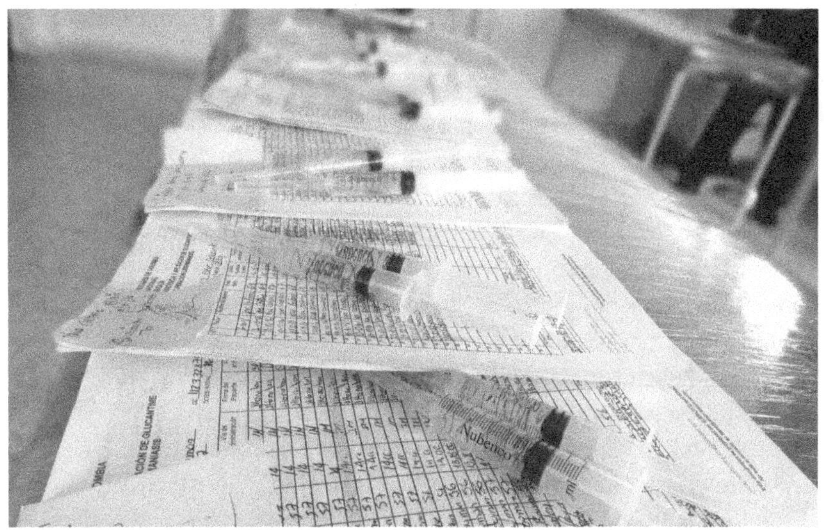

FIGURE 3.2. Pairs of syringes filled with Glucantime. Photo by Lina Pinto-García.

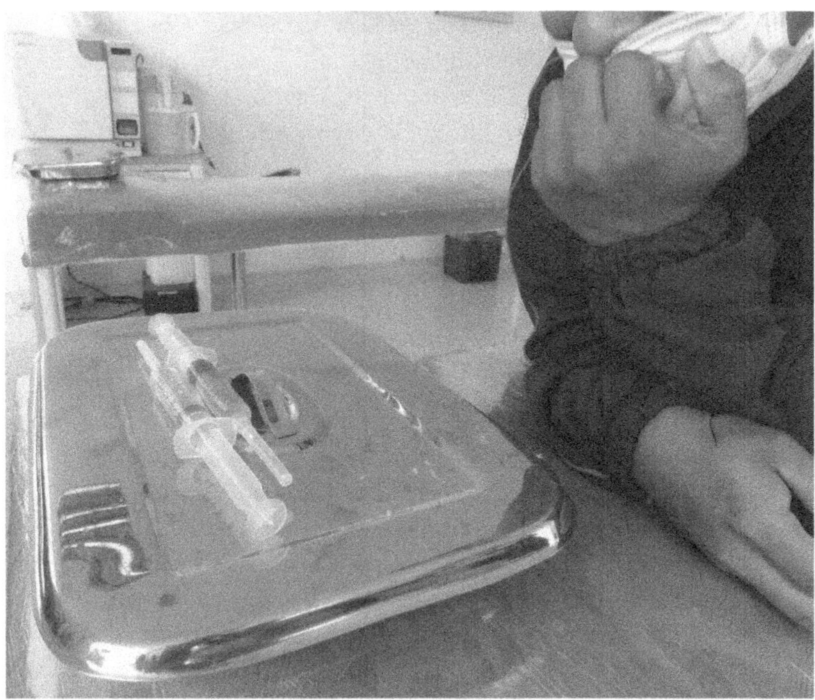

FIGURE 3.3. A soldier with leishmaniasis looks anxiously at the Glucantime injections that are about to be administered to him. Photo by Lina Pinto-García.

Carolina, the chief nurse, prepared the drug doses according to each soldier's weight.[1] She left pairs of syringes on each soldier's record form and lined them up along an empty stretcher (fig. 3.2). Marisol took García's two syringes and placed them on a stainless steel box resting on the stretcher's cushion (fig. 3.3). She asked him to lower his pants, then disinfected both of his buttocks with a cotton ball soaked in alcohol. After identifying a not-quite-sore spot with the tip of her fingers, she injected the medication slowly, deep into the muscle. García's face reddened as he bit the sleeve of his sweatshirt in an effort to withstand the pain. Marisol injected the contents of the second syringe. Finally, after one or two very distressing minutes, García let out a deep sigh, pulled up his pants, and stood up grimacing, making gestures and sounds of pain and discomfort. He rubbed his buttocks with both hands and, clutching the leg of the stretcher, he squatted several times. García still needed to undergo seven out of twenty days of injection treatment. He signed the notebook in which Marisol registered all the procedures she performed, thanked her unenthusiastically, and left the room.

In a span of roughly two hours, this process was repeated with seventy young soldiers. By the end, a bin lined with red plastic and filled with hundreds of empty Glucantime ampoules evidenced the mass treatment and intoxication that had taken place there (fig. 3.4). The CRL follows the same procedure every day of the year, adhering to a rigorous system of inscription, data collection, and accountability put in place by the Army.

Exceptional from every vantage point, the CRL is unlike most other comparable medical infrastructures, designed solely to treat cutaneous leishmaniasis on a massive scale among a highly specific male population. The facility relies on a clinical practice standard to systematically administer Glucantime using a mass-treatment approach designed for efficiency, adhering to a specific sequence of steps. The medical and disciplinary procedures involved, followed with military rigor, cannot be found anywhere else—not even in other clinical facilities of the Colombian Army where leishmaniasis is treated. Some of these procedures include conducting several laboratory tests and electrocardiograms before, during, and after the treatment; the highly organized administration of Glucantime systemically; curative practices that help the lesion to scar; and physiotherapy sessions to alleviate the swelling in the buttocks and reduce the accumulation of Glucantime in the muscle fibers that results from multiple injections over the course of twenty days. Why was this specialized clinical facility created? When did the Colombian Army decide to create this particular infrastructure, and how does it work?

In this chapter, I explore a crucial moment in the history of the *maraña* formed by leishmaniasis and the armed conflict—the context in which this

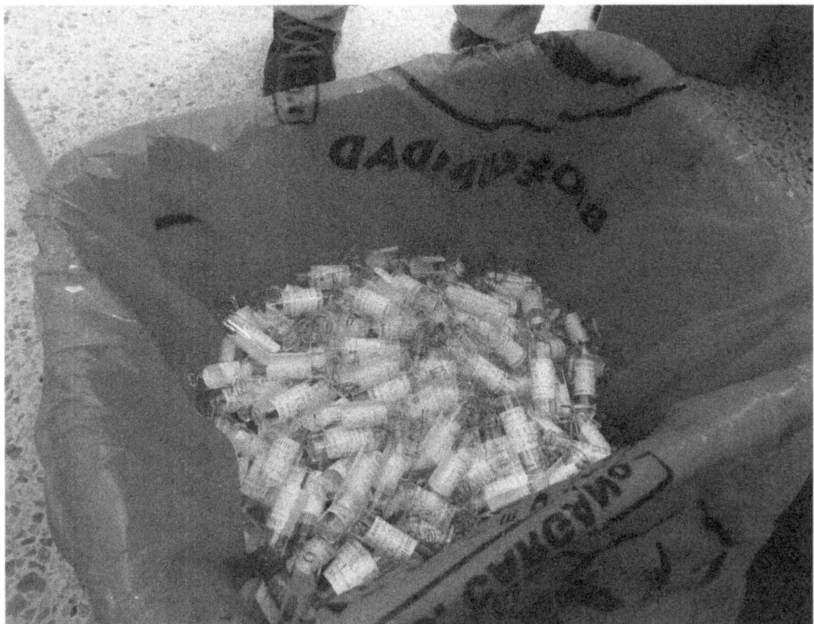

FIGURE 3.4. A trash can full of empty Glucantime ampoules after a single day of leishmaniasis treatment at CRL. Photo by Lina Pinto-García.

disease became a strategy and security problem for the Army in the state war against guerrillas. I focus on the measures adopted by the military once the state realized that maintaining its military force largely depended on healing soldiers with leishmaniasis lesions so they could return to battle. To solve this overwhelming problem, the Army adopted the civilian regulations and technological tools made available by MinSalud. In addition, administering Glucantime treatment and facilitating lesion healing necessitated the establishment of an unparalleled clinic and the development of innovative health practices unique to the military.

During the war, when human resources were at a premium because of the detrimental effects caused by leishmaniasis, keeping soldiers available for the war became a military mission assigned to medical and military personnel in charge of treating leishmaniasis in the Army. I show that in the mid-2000s, warfare strategies and technoscience were engaged in an intense process of mutually shaping and reinforcing where pharmaceuticals, infrastructures, health care practices, and a clinical practice standard were crucial to continuing the war. Since then, leishmaniasis rehabilitation has become integral to military medicine in Colombia more for its capacity to bring soldiers back to duty rather than back to health. War and technoscience have developed simultaneously and reciprocally to sustain the state's ability to fight against guerrilla organizations. In particular, the extensive use of antileishmanial drugs and the Army's adoption of a civilian clinical practice standard to put soldiers back on the front lines is a reminder that "our technologies mirror our societies" (Bijker and Law 1994, 3). A society at war shapes and is shaped by war technologies, which include much more than weapons. This chapter describes how pharmaceutical technological objects have been part of the material, social, and moral landscapes of warfare in Colombia and are elements that lend even more intricacy and complexity to the *maraña*.

A Note on Soldiers of the Colombian Army

According to World Bank data, Colombia has the highest military expenditure as a percentage of GDP in Latin America and the second-largest armed forces after Brazil (IISS 2019). Nonetheless, the relative size of the armed forces to the population is very different in these two countries. Colombia has forty-eight million people, less than a quarter of the Brazilian population. However, while Brazil has sixteen military members for every ten thousand inhabitants, Colombia has sixty-one (IISS 2019). Despite the signing of the 2016 peace accords, internal security remains a priority for the Colombian Army. In particular, counterinsurgency and counternarcotics operations continue to be the main focus of military action.

Colombian law asserts that every man is obliged to report to the Army and "define his military situation" from the moment he reaches the legal age of eighteen. Secondary school students who are eighteen or older can delay this obligation until they obtain their school diploma. For those declared *aptos* (fit), "the government may establish different modalities to meet the obligation of compulsory military service" (Ejército Nacional, n.d.-b).[2] Young men who have finished secondary school enlist as *soldados bachilleres* (secondary school graduate soldiers) for twelve months.[3] Those who did not go to school, which is often the case in rural areas of Colombia, were until very recently recruited as *soldados regulares* (regular soldiers) for a longer period of military service lasting between eighteen and twenty-four months. Because this policy discriminated mainly against rural youth who were not guaranteed the right to education under the constitution, the Constitutional Court established in February 2020 that compulsory military service must last twelve months, regardless of a person's education (J. Rodríguez 2020).

If *soldados regulares* and *soldados bachilleres* manage to stay alive and "successfully" complete their military service, they receive a reservist card, better known in Colombia as the *libreta militar*. This document proves that a man over eighteen has fulfilled his legal obligation of "defining his military situation." Young men from families that can pay for the *libreta* to avoid the military service—a payment the Army calls the military compensation quota—usually do so. That quota is equivalent to 1 percent of the family's assets plus 60 percent of the family's monthly income divided by the number of siblings enrolled in educational institutions (Ejército Nacional, n.d.-a). However, low-income families have generally been unable to afford this payment, especially before some reforms to the conscription process were introduced by the 2017 Recruitment Law. Their children are usually the ones who end up fighting in the war, swelling the Army ranks.

The *libreta* is a secondary identification for young men in Colombia. Until the end of 2014, students needed it to graduate from any university (RCN 2014). Even today, the *libreta* is necessary to work in the public sector and some companies, and it functions as a protective document against forced recruitment in military raids (locally known as *batidas*), which young men still fear and experience despite their prohibition in 2011 (*El Espectador* 2019; *El Tiempo* 2013). Although the situation has slightly improved in recent years thanks to courageous civil society initiatives[4] and laws and rulings passed during the peace negotiations in Havana (see Herrera Durán 2015), forced Army recruitment continues to affect several young men from marginalized backgrounds (Defensoría del Pueblo 2014). Moreover, this compulsory enlistment continues to exacerbate the structural conditions of inequality that force the poorest people into providing labor and cannon fodder to the Colombian armed conflict (see Serrano 2017).

Besides *soldados regulares* and *soldados bachilleres*, the lowest ranks of the Army are made up of so-called *soldados profesionales* (professional soldiers). In 2000, the Army established the Training School for Professional Soldiers (Escuela de Soldados Profesionales del Ejército Nacional, hereafter ESPRO) to train soldiers more efficiently and increase the recruitment of young men by offering more attractive working conditions. While the number of *soldados bachilleres* in the Army has decreased substantially since 2000, the number of professional soldiers went from 40,918 in 2000 to 75,144 in 2006 (Avila 2019, 288). Today, professional soldiers represent the vast majority of those on the front line. The ESPRO recruits men between eighteen and twenty-three who have finished their mandatory military service—but not necessarily secondary school—and want to join the Army as professional soldiers. They have to pay a fee (about 175 US dollars) to join the ESPRO and complete sixteen weeks of training to be called a professional soldier (ESPRO 2019, n.d.). As of January 22, 2019, this military school had trained 86,107 people (ESPRO, n.d.). A professional soldier receives a monthly salary equivalent to the current legal minimum wage increased by 40 percent, which in 2023 corresponds to 1,624,000 Colombian pesos (about 385 US dollars).

Since 1976, both men and women are part of the Colombian Army. However, until 2009, military women could only occupy low-profile administrative positions, and no command or combat responsibilities were assigned to them. This situation started to change in 2011 when forty-eight women became officers with the rank of *subtenientes* (second lieutenants) (Ejército Nacional 2013); however, the Army remains a male-dominated institution. Women occupy barely 10 percent of the military forces (Palomino 2023). In April 2018, it was announced for the first time in history that a woman, Angie Carolina Cely Abril, would be part of the front line of combat (Ejército Nacional 2018). Apart from her and four other women, the first line is made up exclusively of men, and male officers disproportionately dominate positions of power in the chain of command (Barreto-Romero, Ortíz-Forero, and Cely 2020). After twenty years of accepting only men for military service, the Army received 1,296 women in 2023. However, they do not serve in combat roles (Palomino 2023).

So far, I have used the word *soldier* as a broad term to refer to male members of the Army. Although I continue to use this term in that general way, especially in this and the next chapter, I must clarify several points. Leishmaniasis is a disease that only affects troops in forward areas—in the jungle, in locations the military call *el área* or *el área de operaciones* (the area of operations). This indicates, first, that there are no female Army members with leishmaniasis, which explains why the words *he*, *men*, *servicemen*, and *manpower* abound in this book about war and leishmaniasis. Second, high-ranking officers (*mayores*, *coroneles*, and *generales*) are never present in the area of operations.[5] Thus, those who contract the disease are exclusively men in the lowest ranks (*regular*, *bachiller*, and *profesional* soldiers) and their commanders: the subofficers (*cabos* and *sargentos*) and low-ranking officers (*subtenientes*, *tenientes*, and *capitanes*). Because they represent the majority of military personnel in the area of operations, soldiers—especially professional soldiers—are most frequently affected by the disease. For instance, in 2016, soldiers made up 90.7 percent of all leishmaniasis cases treated at the CRL, and 80.8 percent of them were professional soldiers. In contrast, subofficers and officers represented only 8 percent and 1.4 percent, respectively. Thus, using the word *soldier* also emphasizes that it is these young men in the lower tier of the military hierarchy and at the bottom of the social pyramid both inside and outside the Army who are predominantly affected by leishmaniasis.

Leishmaniasis and the State War against Guerrillas

After graduating from high school in the late 1990s, Major Saúl Chacón joined the Escuela Militar de Cadetes General José María Córdova to become an officer in the Colombian Army. In 2002, he began his military career as a platoon commander in the northern part of the country. A year and a half later, he was transferred to a *batallón de contraguerrilla* (counterinsurgency battalion) in northwestern Colombia, an area heavily affected by the armed conflict. Although the work was tremendously exhausting and dangerous, Major Chacón told me those were his best years in the Army. "I experienced the best moments of camaraderie. A very strong camaraderie is formed among the personnel because you go through so many intense situations. The people I met at that time are still my friends to this day," he told me, smiling. Leishmaniasis, he recalled, was one of the many difficulties he had to face there for the first time. While discussing what this disease represented for members of the Army, he explained: "As a military man, you knew you were going to be affected by leishmaniasis—at some point it's going to be your turn. In some places, it's so frequent that it's like getting a cold. I mean, if you didn't get leishmaniasis [in those areas], you weren't there. If your body wasn't marked somewhere [by leishmaniasis], you weren't there." Although leishmaniasis has historically affected a wide variety of people who live close to and interact with the forests, its prevalence among Army members is particularly high. Of all the infectious and vector-borne diseases, soldiers are most affected by leishmaniasis—far more than dengue, malaria, chikungunya, Zika, yellow fever, and Chagas disease (Ministerio de Defensa et al. 2017). The military is one of the most vulnerable populations when it comes to leishmaniasis and, according to official data, has shown the highest incidence rate in Colombia (Patino et al. 2017). In fact, leishmaniasis is a disease inherent to soldiering, part of the challenges of the military role in Colombia, a physical reminder of the military's connection to the jungle. It would be unusual for a male soldier to have escaped this disease and its treatments during his service.

As I mentioned earlier, with Álvaro Uribe's PSD soldier recruitment increased by 31.6 percent (Leal Buitrago 2011), and the military approach drastically changed from a defensive to an offensive strategy. The Plan Patriota, launched in 2004 as a crucial element of the PSD, was a two-phased military plan that received financial support from the United States and sought to expand military state presence into areas where guerrilla organizations were traditionally dominant. The PSD, but especially the Plan Patriota, represented an unprecedented change in terms of military strategy and scale of war. While the first phase of this plan focused on regaining full control of the areas surrounding Bogotá, the capital, the second sought to recover the territorial domination that guerrilla groups had established in rural areas in southern parts of the country (*Semana* 2006; Ruiz 2004). Thus, soldiers were forced to enter the jungle in large numbers and stay there for several months to maintain sustained military pressure in the form of harassment and persecution of guerrillas, especially of the FARC. Guerrilla organizations responded by deploying antipersonnel land mines, which led to an average of 764 mortal (20 percent) and nonmortal (80 percent) victims every year between 2000 and 2010, most of them (68 percent) part of the Public Force.[6]

At that point, land mines—but also leishmaniasis—became critical obstacles in the state war against guerrillas. As Major Chacón told me, in some areas of the country such as Urabá,[7] soldiers had "two options, either leaving with incomplete legs [due to land mines] or leaving with the mark of leishmaniasis; if you were in Urabá, it was certain you were going to get leishmaniasis." Yet, while the impact of land mines during this period is well documented and understood (see CNMH and Fundación Prolongar 2017), there is much less awareness of the dangers and consequences of leishmaniasis and its pharmaceutical treatment during the most intense years of the war.

As I related in chapter 1, between 2003 and 2006, the largest leishmaniasis outbreak recorded in Colombia occurred in Chaparral, Tolima. In the mid-2000s, newspapers reported the unusual rise of leishmaniasis cases and attributed the main cause to the increase in state combatants entering areas with a high risk of disease transmission (see *El Tiempo* 2004a, 2006; Quintero 2005). Indeed, leishmaniasis became the leading reason for removing soldiers from combat. Furthermore, the success of the Plan Patriota was repeatedly questioned given the high number of casualties[8] in the Army, not because of combat injuries but from other causes such as leishmaniasis (see *El Tiempo* 2004b, 2004c; Leal Buitrago 2006). In 2005, when there were 178,000 active members in the Army (IISS 2005), land mines and leishmaniasis were the leading causes of men's withdrawal from military duties, resulting in nearly ten thousand casualties in one year—many more than those caused by direct combat (Bedoya Lima 2006b, 2006a; *El Tiempo* 2005a; US Embassy in Colombia 2006a). In fact, in 2005 and 2006, there was a spike in both leishmaniasis cases and land mine victims among Public Force members (fig. 3.5). However, while there were 755 and 790 victims of land mines in the Public Force in 2005 and 2006, respectively, the Army registered 9,800 and 9,623 cases of leishmaniasis in those same two years.[9]

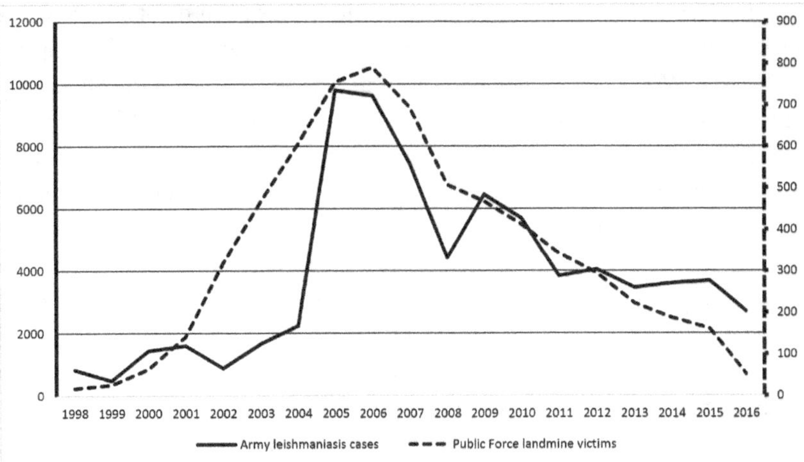

FIGURE 3.5. In this graph, cases of leishmaniasis in the Army are represented by a black line, and fatal and nonfatal land mine casualties in the Public Force (Army, Air Force, Navy, and Police) are depicted with a dashed black line. It is important to note that each plotted line uses a different scale. If the same scale were applied to both, the line representing land mine casualties would appear almost flat due to the significantly higher number of leishmaniasis cases compared to land mine casualties. The 1998–2003 leishmaniasis figures, which include both cutaneous and mucosal forms of the disease, come from an Army document (DGSM 2010); the 2004–2016 figures, which also include cutaneous and mucosal leishmaniasis cases, were provided by the Army at my request. The 1998–2016 land mine figures, which include all Public Force victims of both land mines and unexploded ordnance, come from the Directorate for Integral Action Against Antipersonnel Mines (DAICMA) database. Although the DAICMA database does not discriminate among institutions of the Public Force, members of the Army are the most numerous victims of land mines among the four state armed forces (see CNMH and Fundación Prolongar 2017).

References: CNMH and Fundación Prolongar. 2017. La Guerra Escondida: Minas Antipersonal y Remanentes Explosivos En Colombia. Bogotá: CNMH. DGSM. 2010. "Directiva Permanente No. 143581."

Thus, in that period, the disease affected 5.5 percent of the Army each year. These men were not at the front line of combat where they were needed and expected to be; instead, they spent their time in military clinical facilities receiving treatment and waiting for their ulcers to heal. Despite the fact that the annual incidence of leishmaniasis among servicemen gradually decreased in the years after 2006, it returned to comparable 2004 rates (2,241 cases) only in 2016 (2,699 cases) when the peace deal with the FARC was reached.

Several scholars have highlighted the importance of insect vectors and the diseases they transmit in shaping political and historical events in significant ways. In particular, the role of mosquitoes in the transmission of potentially lethal diseases such as malaria and yellow fever has been pivotal in conflicts such as the American Civil War, Cuba's battle for independence from Spain, and World War II (A. M. Bell 2010; Espinosa 2009; Slater 2009). "Mercenary mosquitoes mustered armies of pestilence and stalked battlefields across the globe, often deciding the outcome of game-changing wars" (Winegard 2019, 4). The case of leishmaniasis and the Colombian armed conflict is unusual because, unlike these other diseases, leishmaniasis is not fatal, and the vector is not the all-too-familiar mosquito. Studying leishmaniasis reveals how nonlethal infectious diseases transmitted by carriers other than mosquitoes can have an equally significant impact on the course of war and other events of political, social, and historical importance.

How has leishmaniasis posed challenges for the Army? First, leishmaniasis has created a significant financial burden for the state in general and the Army in particular. Keeping a man out of combat is costly. It is also expensive to get him out of the jungle because the usual way out is by helicopter. The costs associated with the diagnosis, treatment, and medical follow-up are also high, as well as returning a recovered soldier to his military unit and then to the area of operations. As Timothy Winegard crudely reminds us, "a sick soldier is more taxing to the military machine than a dead one. Not only do they need to be replaced but they also continue to consume valuable resources" (Winegard 2019, 4). In the Army, leishmaniasis is regarded as an *enfermedad profesional* (occupational disease), which means that the circumstances under which a soldier is infected occur "in the service, for cause and reason thereof."[10] Defining leishmaniasis as an occupational disease acknowledges that it is a consequence of the labor performed by military personnel while on duty, making the Army health subsystem responsible for all leishmaniasis-related health care services required by a member of the military (see DGSM 2008). This responsibility entails spending scarce resources, both financial and medical. According to a CRL staff member, a soldier staying at the CRL in 2016 represented approximately COP 110,000 (about USD 35) per day for the Army. As an Army colonel physician explained: "That person stops working for at least three months. However, we must continue paying his salary, food, health, and accommodation. Then, this represents a detriment for the Army." Additionally, the Army provides compensation to its members for disabilities and decreased ability to work. As I explain in more detail in chapter 4, the Army compensates men for the scars and other consequences related to leishmaniasis treatment. Given the high prevalence of the disease among soldiers, these compensations also imply high charges for the Army.

Despite being the less expensive pharmaceutical for treating leishmaniasis, Glucantime ampoules are nevertheless relatively costly. And although the Army is responsible for the medical care of its leishmaniasis patients, it is important to mention that, while the military recognizes leishmaniasis as an occupational illness, it is not the Ministry of Defense but the Ministry of Health that pays for antileishmanial treatment for all Army personnel. In other words, the budgetary state allocation for public health—not for defense—has been paying to treat a disease soldiers acquire while on duty—while "defending the nation," as the military likes to say. Between 1997 and 2017, the Ministry of Health spent more than 17 million USD on the purchase of Glucantime ampoules, many of which were allocated to the Army.[11] While the price of Glucantime ampoules significantly decreased in 2010 when Colombia started acquiring the drug through the PAHO Strategic Fund, purchasing Glucantime has represented a considerable expense for the state and a substantial profit for the pharmaceutical company Sanofi.[12]

Secondly but even more importantly, leishmaniasis has been a security concern and strategic problem in the state war against the guerrillas. In the mid-2000s, when large numbers of soldiers penetrated the forests and stayed there for months seeking to expel guerrillas, leishmaniasis affected troops in massive proportions, forcing commanders to regularly remove men from areas of operation. Thus, leishmaniasis jeopardized the Army's performance and its capacity to maintain control over territories it had fought for and conquered.

Army officer Camilo Bernal explained the situation further to me. He became an officer in the early 2000s, which means that he enlisted during the peak of the war and was permanently deployed to forward areas—in the jungle—until 2008. He told me he had been very lucky to survive those military operations and without losing any of his limbs to antipersonnel mines. Recalling the change in military strategy that resulted from Uribe's PSD and how leishmaniasis was experienced in the Army at that time, Camilo told me the following:

> One thing is to go [to the jungle], look for the guerrillas, and go back. Another thing is to go and stay there, maintain presence. At that moment [mid-2000s], the disease affected the [military] force a lot. For example, let's say you were going to deploy a battalion of 240 men in a certain area. Two months later you had 180 men, four months later you had 50 men. You didn't have a battalion anymore. Then, leishmaniasis becomes a problem, even a security problem, because you can't maintain [presence] and you have to move back, take people

> out. You lose what you had gained, you lose the territorial position. More than a common disease . . . leishmaniasis, for us, became a problem at the strategic level because it affected us so much that the strength capacity of the Army decreased. I mean, [military] units were diminished, completely segregated due to leishmaniasis.

At that time, leishmaniasis was no longer considered a minor health issue for the military. Instead, its effects came to be seen as a serious manpower problem that led to strategic and security problems. During that crucial period of the Colombian war, the Army quickly realized that maintaining the state military force depended largely on healing soldiers of their leishmaniasis lesions so they could return to the conflict. Thus, military medicine, particularly the pharmacological treatment of leishmaniasis, became crucial to the management of manpower resources in Colombia. In fact, leishmaniasis is the only disease for which the Army established a specialized clinical facility dedicated exclusively to the medical management of soldier-patients affected by it. Moreover, at the primary unit for medical care and rehabilitation for soldiers of the Colombian Army, the Military Health Battalion (BASAN) in Bogotá, leishmaniasis is the only disease that defines and categorizes one of the five *compañías* (military units) that make up the battalion. The other four *compañías*—orthopedics, internal medicine, amputations, and a special company of orthopedics and amputations—are not identified by a particular disease, which highlights the significance of leishmaniasis to the Army (see Carmona Lozano 2016).

In his analysis of the links among HIV/AIDS, war, and security, Fernando Serrano-Amaya (2013) discusses how, in the late 1990s and early 2000s, this infectious disease was redefined as a central security concern at the national, regional, and international levels, especially in relation to sub-Saharan African countries experiencing internal conflicts. Understanding securitization as "a speech act by which an issue is constructed as a matter of security" (2013, 316), Serrano-Amaya asserts that framing HIV/AIDS as a top-down, state-centered security concern led to the widespread but unexamined assumption that armed conflict causes the propagation of HIV/AIDS. Moreover, "the securitization of HIV/AIDS incorporated a logic of 'threat-defense' to the management of the epidemic" that focused on the military's attention and response while neglecting the vulnerabilities of the civilian population to the disease (2013, 319). Insofar as the disease posed a threat to army members and military operations, framing HIV/AIDS as a security issue led to prioritizing treatment and prevention programs focused on preserving soldiers' health, combat capability, and national defense (Serrano-Amaya 2013; O'Manique 2005).

Although there is no official discourse on leishmaniasis as a security problem in Colombia, this chapter shows how, in practice, the state prioritized the military regarding the rise of leishmaniasis cases from the mid-2000s onward. Regarding leishmaniasis as an obstacle to the development of military operations that jeopardized the PSD's achievements, the state focused its efforts to combat the disease on the Army. Similar to the securitization of HIV/AIDS, the securitization of leishmaniasis was reflected in the military's prevention, diagnosis, and treatment strategies, none of which were extended to civilians, let alone the insurgent population that remained hidden in the forests.

To address the severe shortage of human resources caused by leishmaniasis, the pharmaceutical management of this disease became a key part of rehabilitative practices within the Army and was an indispensable component of the state war against guerrilla organizations. In other words, leishmaniasis health care became institutionally subordinated to the war apparatus. This development is part of a long-existing trend in state power, which became particularly conspicuous after Europe's colonial expansion in the early nineteenth century (Worboys 2003). Protecting troops and administrators from the diseases of colonized territories was a major challenge and primary objective of the colonial mission. Thus, at the end of the nineteenth century, colonial medicine was established through institutions dedicated to studying so-called tropical diseases, training medical personnel in the emerging specialty of tropical medicine and hygiene, and developing technologies to protect the military and other populations whose health was vital to the advancement of the colonial project. While the use of quinine against malaria was crucial to the European colonization of Africa (Curtin 1989) and the triumph of the Union in the American Civil War (A. M. Bell 2010), the development of chloroquine was equally significant in the Second World War, protecting millions of US Army soldiers from the debilitating and potentially fatal effects of malaria (Slater 2009). As I explained in the introduction, before the outbreak of World War II, France purchased antileishmanial drugs from Germany. Thus, the development of Glucantime resulted from the lack of antileishmanial treatments among Allied soldiers during the war. Glucantime, as I will explain further, has also played an important role in the management of human resources during the war in Colombia.

The important position held by the medical and especially pharmaceutical management of leishmaniasis in the Colombian Army is similar to the significant role played by rehabilitation and the specialty of orthopedics during the First World War, especially in Germany (Linker 2011; Perry 2014). In a comparative historical work, Anderson and Perry (2014) argue that, unlike Great Britain, Germany had no dominions or colonies from which to recruit replacements for those wounded in the Great War. Thus, "the military turned to the nation's orthopaedists and demanded that they speed up and maximize further the recovery and service potential of Germany's severely wounded soldiers" (2014, 241). The goal of German rehabilitation was to address its manpower shortage by returning disabled soldiers to the field of battle. Similarly, since the mid-2000s, leishmaniasis rehabilitation became integral to military medicine in Colombia because it allowed soldiers to return to the front lines. Thus, keeping human resources available for the war became a mission assigned to medical workers and military personnel in charge of treating and healing leishmaniasis in the Army.

Anthropologists have drawn attention to the use of pharmaceuticals in the military to maintain operational readiness in contemporary conflicts. For example, Jocelyn Lim Chua (2018) has studied the prescription of psychiatric drugs among members of the US Army, an increasingly common and accepted practice since the mid-2000s (see also Gray 2015; Howell 2011). According to Chua, the fact that the so-called Global War on Terrorism relies on a completely voluntary force has necessitated a psychopharmaceutical management of limited human resources to ensure readiness for war and a swift return to combat. Importantly, Chua examines the movement of psychoactive medicines into combat settings and explores how the effects of these drugs change when they are prescribed and used in the context of war. In this environment, Chua asserts, medications are strategically used not to restore soldiers to complete health but to heal them just enough to allow them to return to fighting. Drug treatment allows soldiers to be returned to the same conditions of suffering, violence, and death that made them sick in the first place. The use of these technologies results in "a perversion of the therapeutic value of drugs [that] highlights the tensions of medicalized efforts to keep soldiers healthy and alive in and for war" (Chua 2018, 23).

As Chua points out, the delivery of pharmaceuticals into military bodies serves as a valuable way to consider the soldier's exceptional biopolitical condition. In his ethnography of the daily lives of soldiers involved in war-making at one of the largest military posts in the US, Kenneth T. MacLeish (2013) carefully explores the ways in which the status and bodily experience of the soldier are exceptional. He writes that the soldier is unique because he has the power to kill but is also systematically exposed to harm and the possibility of death. As such, he is both the instrument and the object of state-imposed violence. Moreover, "he is the subject of extensive measures to protect and maintain life, to keep him alive and able to continue working, fighting, and killing effectively, a biopolitical subject not merely kept from dying but also made to live" (MacLeish 2015, 15–16). By understanding the soldier's body as the most basic war material—the crucial piece in whose absence war simply does not happen—MacLeish recognizes that when a soldier's body is incapable of recovery, it is discarded and replaced. In his words, "The body's unruly matter is war's most necessary and most necessarily expendable raw material" (MacLeish 2013, 11). Thus, instead of focusing on restoring a soldier's health, the purpose of health care under military jurisdiction is to ensure that the soldier can return to the battlefield for as long as they are deemed valuable (Thomson 1998). In his study of the development of enhancement biotechnologies to produce "supersoldiers" in the US military, Andrew Bickford (2020) conducts a similar analysis. He claims that the military and civilian medical professions differ in their definition and practice of health care. In the military, health is mobilized and instrumentalized as "a conception that harnesses rather than explicitly heals, one that sees biology as something to overcome and manipulate in order to make it useful" (2020, 9). In this sense, the soldier's body is a material problem, one that requires relentless efforts on the military's part to "extract as much labor power—or 'combat capability'—from the soldier as possible" (2020, 8).

Drawing inspiration from this research, I show how leishmaniasis health care in the Colombian Army is shaped to respond primarily to the manpower demands of the military rather than to the medical needs of the soldier with leishmaniasis. By examining the institutional management of this disease, I further expand on the conditions under which the Army established a clinical infrastructure devoted exclusively to leishmaniasis. I also highlight the role that pharmaceuticals, a clinical practice guideline, and novel health care practices have played in healing soldiers' bodies only to return them to the battlefield—to the very same conditions that made them sick in the first place. I explore what happens to these technologies when they are used in a military setting and required to maintain the Army's combat capability under a permanent state of war.

The Pharmaceuticalization of War in the Army

As I have explained, the state's governance of leishmaniasis in Colombia is pharmaceuticalized and centered on Glucantime. In other words, the public health strategy for dealing with leishmaniasis revolves almost entirely around pharmaceuticals, and Glucantime is the primary drug administered to those patients who can access the diagnosis and treatment. Likewise, the Army has acknowledged the potential of this drug to solve the manpower shortage caused by leishmaniasis. As such, two essential aspects of the *pharmaceuticalization of war* have been the Army's extensive use of Glucantime and the concentration of most of the institutional management of the military personnel affected by the disease on this medicine. The connection between war and pharmaceutical regimes is evident in the Army's use of Glucantime to solve the manpower crisis produced by leishmaniasis.

Even before the mid-2000s leishmaniasis epidemic, the Army's response to the disease was already focused on Glucantime. At the time, however, it might be several weeks before a soldier diagnosed with leishmaniasis could obtain the drug. Additionally, the treatment was not medically supervised, and laboratory tests were not performed to monitor the soldier-patient's health before, during, and after the therapeutic process. The doses of Glucantime were not necessarily those recommended by health professionals, and servicemen rarely used all the ampoules prescribed—once they saw that their lesion had healed, many of them interrupted the treatment. Moreover, Glucantime was often administered in the jungle where the fighting occurred without any medical assistance beyond what a soldier trained as a combat nurse could provide. In short, the Army's management of leishmaniasis was not regulated or standardized by any protocol, and Glucantime circulated freely among its members. The persistence of skin ulcers despite Glucantime treatment, medical complications (e.g., infection at the injection site, hepatitis, nephritis, or cardiotoxicity), and the deaths of several soldiers resulted from a lack of regulations for leishmaniasis treatment. Also, the Glucantime ampoules allocated to the Army by MinSalud were easily stolen by corrupt military personnel to meet the needs of leishmaniasis sufferers outside of the Army, such as members of guerrilla and paramilitary groups.

Faced with this critical situation, the Army Health Office (Dirección de Sanidad Militar, henceforth DISAN) determined that soldiers with the disease had to be evacuated from the areas of operation and moved to one of the few military hospitals or clinical facilities where the administration of Glucantime was regulated according to MinSalud's clinical practice guidelines (CPG). Measures were taken to prevent theft by tightly controlling the ampoules' movement within the Army. The CPG, first created in 2000 and updated in 2010, 2018, and 2023, has been used by the Army to institutionalize, systematize, and enforce a therapeutic approach to leishmaniasis based on the massive administration of Glucantime at a dose of 20 mg/kg per day for twenty consecutive days (twenty-eight days for cases of mucosal leishmaniasis). The Army refers to the appropriation and implementation of the

CPG in military clinical facilities in the mid-2000s as the Institutional Leishmaniasis Program.

In addition, the Army implemented various strategies to prevent the disease among troops stationed in forested areas. The DISAN initiated leishmaniasis health campaigns so that servicemen, despite their obligatory long-term exposure to the disease, would take active measures to avoid contracting it. They were ordered to keep their bodies completely covered by their uniform—sleeves and pants never rolled up. Likewise, a contingency plan was implemented for the military use of *toldillos* (mosquito nets), repellents, and uniforms that were saturated with an insecticide called Permethrin (PECET and Fuerzas Militares de Colombia 2005, 38). Not just any repellent was appropriate; it had to be odorless so that troops would not be detected by guerrillas. Thus, the use of unscented repellents with DEET (diethyltoluamide), such as Nopikex and Ultrathon, became mandatory for military personnel.[13] According to classified cables released by WikiLeaks in 2005, "Budget limitations and distribution problems [were] making it hard for the [Colombian] military to obtain [antileishmanial] drugs in sufficient quantities" (US Embassy in Colombia 2005b). Thus, the Colombian government asked the US government to help cover the expenses related to the increasing demand for Glucantime in the Army (US Embassy in Colombia 2005a). However, the United States was unable to provide financial assistance for that purpose because the US Food and Drug Administration had yet to approve a treatment for leishmaniasis.[14] Instead, the US government provided 500,000 USD to the Colombian Army to purchase insect repellents such as DEET and Permethrin (US Embassy in Colombia 2005c).

Although vector-control strategies to prevent or minimize pathogenic interactions between humans and parasite-carrying sandflies are generally not part of the state management of leishmaniasis for nonmilitary populations, the use of mosquito nets and repellents in the Army has not been effective (A. M. González, Solis-Soto, and Radon 2017). I discussed this with soldiers at the CRL, and many of them confirmed that they each receive a bottle of Ultrathon and a mosquito net as part of their equipment. However, even though Ultrathon is mandatory in the jungle, some prefer not to use it because they think it is either ineffective or harmful to the body. For example, Arbeláez, a professional soldier with seven years of Army service, told me that, while patrolling the jungles of Caquetá, his troop came to a forest clearing where the sun's rays shone brightly. Neither he nor his fellow soldiers had been told that Ultrathon burns the skin when exposed to the sun, so they all suffered burns. That experience was enough to keep them from using the repellent again. Soldiers also told me that they usually take tablets of thiamine (vitamin

B1) and so-called garlic pearls so their bodies will emit odors that act as insect repellents. For the same reason, they also eat raw garlic cloves and rub their skin with preparations made from tobacco leaves.

Arbeláez also mentioned that carrying the repellents provided by the Army highlights another problem with these technologies. Equipment weight is such a crucial variable of the Colombian soldier's existence (as well as that of the guerrilla) in the jungle that disagreements often occur because someone—usually the troop commander—is carrying less weight than the rest of the squad. Also, disciplinary punishments can take the form of ordering a soldier to carry extra weight. Thus, deciding whether or not to carry a bottle of repellent is far from being a minor issue. For Arbeláez, the risk of leishmaniasis was less worrisome than the fatigue caused by carrying extra weight that was not absolutely necessary. As for the mosquito net, some soldiers told me that they preferred not to use it. They explained that if at any moment a guerrilla ambush or attack took them by surprise, it would not be very clever to be inside of a net, as it restricts movement and the ability to run away quickly. In other words, soldiers often have to choose between leaving the jungle with leishmaniasis or without their life. Unsurprisingly, most prefer the first alternative.

It is important to reiterate that one of the most significant measures taken by the Army to address the high incidence of leishmaniasis among soldiers was to establish the CRL, an exceptional clinic able to administer Glucantime on a large scale and according to the procedures established by MinSalud's CPG (C. Cruz 2016; Rico Mendoza 2016). The CRL is a military health care facility within the Silva Plazas Battalion—a cavalry military unit with stables and paddocks four hours from Bogotá. It is located in a bucolic landscape of green meadows and mountains where it is possible to hear the nearby neighing of the Army's finest horses. With an average temperature of 14 degrees Celsius throughout the year, the climate is quite cold compared to the warm, humid, and forested areas where soldiers fight guerrillas and get bitten by sandflies. The environmental conditions at the CRL help speed up the soldiers' healing process. Sandflies do not live in this climate, so transmission between infected and uninfected people can be prevented (Medina 2007b, 2007a).

The CRL was built in this location in 2005 because one of the few military dermatologists worked at the Tarqui Artillery Battalion in Sogamoso, less than an hour away from the Silva Plazas Battalion.[15] Overwhelmed by the enormous number of soldiers with leishmaniasis who were being referred to him—mostly from the forested areas where the second phase of the Plan Patriota was being conducted—this dermatologist asked Army commander General Mario Montoya to establish accommodations and a health care facility to treat them. Space was available for such a project at the Silva Plazas

CENTRO NACIONAL
DE REHABILITACION PARA
LEISHMANIASIS
ESTA OBRA SE LLEVO A CABO GRACIAS AL
APOYO PERMANENTE E INCONDICIONAL
DEL SEÑOR GENERAL
MARIO MONTOYA URIBE
COMANDANTE DEL EJERCITO NACIONAL
TENIENDO EN CUENTA EL BIENESTAR Y RECUPERACION DE LOS
HOMBRES QUE SE SACRIFICAN PROFESIONALMENTE POR LA
PAZ DE NUESTRO PAIS SIENDO AFECTADOS
FISICAMENTE POR ESTA ENFERMEDAD
GENERAL MARIO MONTOYA URIBE
COMANDANTE DEL EJERCITO NACIONAL

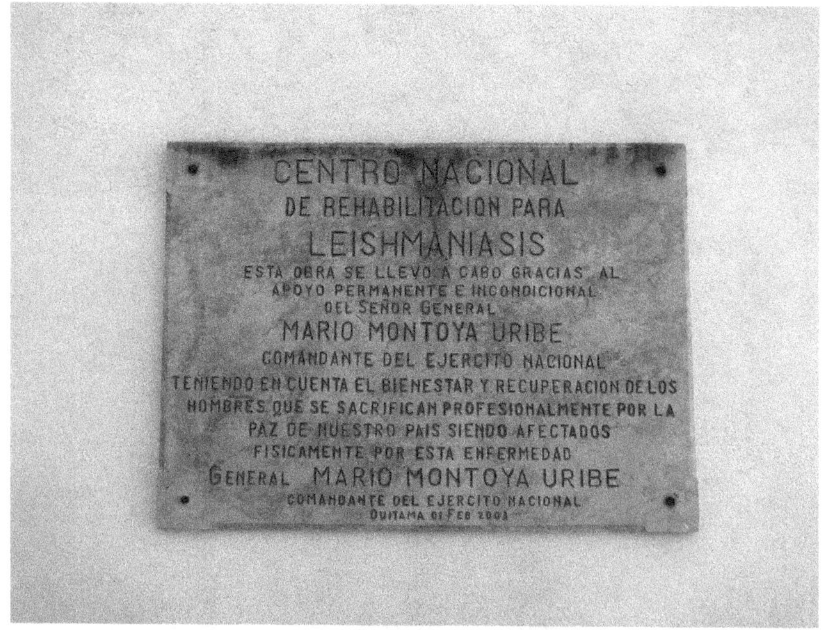

FIGURE 3.6. A carved stone slab commemorating the inauguration of the CRL in 2008. Its inscription says that the "National Center for the Rehabilitation of Leishmaniasis" was established "taking into account the welfare and recovery of the men who professionally make sacrifices for the peace of our country, being physically affected by this disease." Photo by Lina Pinto-García.

Battalion. While it was being built, the CRL operated temporarily in the Tarqui Battalion. In 2008, it was officially inaugurated at its current location (fig. 3.6).

As I stated at the beginning of this chapter, at the CRL, the treatment of leishmaniasis with Glucantime is a carefully designed process under constant medical supervision, carried out by a group of doctors, nurses, and nursing assistants dedicated entirely to the clinical management of this disease. Additionally, only at the CRL are soldier-patients confined to barracks, exempt from physical activities, and able to focus exclusively on their treatment and recovery. Andrea González (the university researcher mentioned in the introduction) used the word *atypical* to describe what she saw at the CRL. She has coordinated multiple biomedical studies on leishmaniasis involving Army personnel. Except for soldiers of the Colombian Army, no one in Colombia—and probably nowhere else in the world—has access to a facility exclusively dedicated to the treatment of leishmaniasis, where Glucantime is administered under the unparalleled conditions found at the CRL. And, I argue, no one outside the Army will ever have access to such a therapeutic experience. Why? Because it is the military regime's exceptional conditions that allow

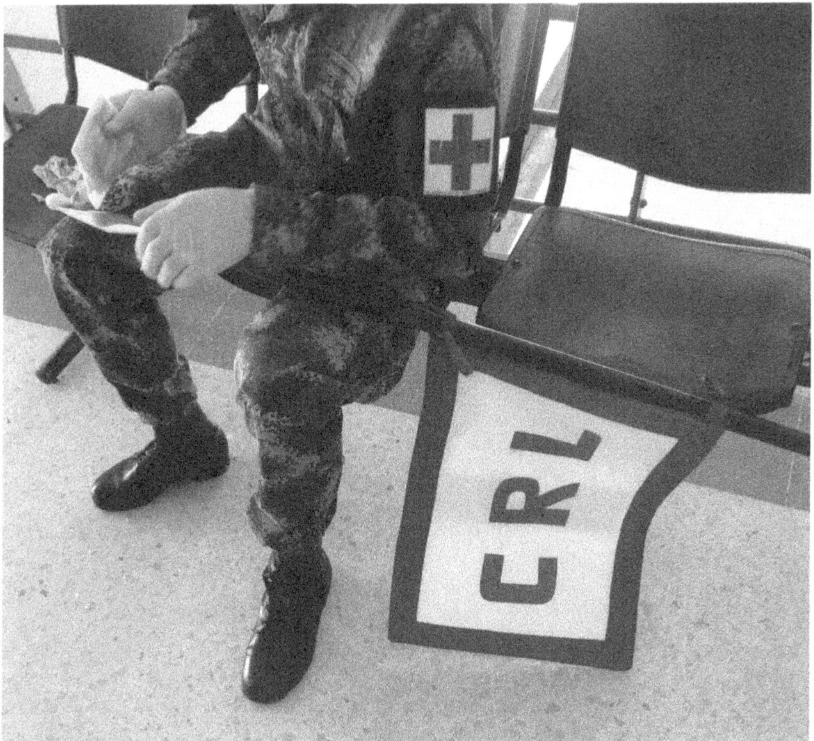

FIGURE 3.7. Military nursing assistant shining the CRL flagpole. Photo by Lina Pinto-García.

for "the unrestrained exercise of medical authority" (Cooter 1990, 152). This is especially evident when we examine the particular way in which the CPG has been appropriated by the Army, which is the focus of the next subsection.

In the Army's view, the CRL epitomizes the medical surveillance conditions necessary to minimize the risks associated with nonrigorous medical practices in navigating leishmaniasis and the toxicity of Glucantime. Consequently, for many members of the military, the Institutional Leishmaniasis Program—and the CRL in particular—is a source of pride, especially for guaranteeing the constant availability of Glucantime and the strict medical control of soldier-patients before, during, and after treatment (fig. 3.7). In fact, members of the Army, some scientists, and government representatives consider the CRL to be a positive legacy of the war and an exemplary model for others in Colombia and internationally. However, as Roger Cooter and Steve Sturdy (1998, 6) remind us, triumphalist narratives about the ways in which war has advanced or favored medicine "are as implicitly militarist as they are naively positivist and partial." This will be particularly evident in the remaining pages of this book.

A CLINICAL PRACTICE GUIDELINE TURNED INTO A MILITARY PROTOCOL

Over the past three decades, evidence-based medicine (EBM) has come to dominate medical discourse and practice on a global scale. Operating on the premise that the best medical care is supported by the review and application of the best available scientific evidence, EBM promotes the ongoing creation of clinical practice guidelines and other medical standards to guide the everyday work of clinicians. However, the widespread adoption of EBM has given rise to intense debate. Advocates defend EBM as a rational and therefore superior approach to medicine whose legitimacy rests on the assumption that scientific evidence is universal and that science is superior to other epistemic practices and forms of knowledge. From this viewpoint, standards are "deemed laudatory; they are something one aspires to live up to" (Timmermans and Epstein 2010, 71). Critics, however, warn of the dangers of EBM expansion, claiming it might turn clinical practice into "cookbook medicine," which would ignore the position of clinical expertise and scientific knowledge production as well as the particular circumstances, needs, and values of each individual patient (Wieringa et al. 2017; Knaapen 2014). Amid this polarized context, others believe that EBM should not automatically be seen as an inherently good or bad paradigm shift. Drawing inspiration from science and technology studies (STS) scholarship, they call on social scientists to favor empirically based research to understand how medical standards are produced, circulate, and work within particular institutional and clinical settings, leading to context-specific consequences (Mykhalovskiy and Weir 2004).

Although every standard specifies a series of actions organized in the form of a "script," Stefan Timmermans and Steven Epstein (2010) have argued that the implementation of clinical practice guidelines resists standardization and is highly dependent on the localized ways in which clinicians use them to make medical decisions. After all, clinical practice guidelines are a set of *recommendations* for the treatment and care of specific health conditions and diseases. Although health care workers are advised to follow them, they can also choose to ignore a particular recommendation based on their medical judgment regarding a specific patient. Usually, "individual clinical autonomy takes precedence over the normative and prescriptive aspect of the guidelines" (Timmermans and Berg 2003, 94). Moreover, tweaking, subverting, or circumventing standards seem necessary to making these documents work as intended. As such, "the trick in standardization appears to be to find a balance between flexibility and rigidity and to trust users with the right amount of agency to keep a standard sufficiently uniform for the task at hand" (Timmermans and Epstein 2010, 81). From this perspective, the ideal clinical practice guideline is one that is flexible and provides options to medical practitioners rather than limiting them to just one course of action.

But what happens when a clinical practice guideline is implemented in an environment characterized by authoritarian rigidity, an undisputable hierarchy, and a reliance on written protocols that must be strictly adhered to in order to avoid disciplinary prosecution? In other words, how does a medical standard work in an exceptional context such as a military clinic? And what if health professionals do not have the tools to reinterpret or adjust the standard because they have never faced the health condition in question before?

MinSalud's CPG for leishmaniasis seeks to standardize how leishmaniasis cases are managed everywhere in Colombia, regardless of the location and the patient. As a guideline, the CPG's recommendations are meant to inform but not necessarily determine the clinical management of leishmaniasis patients. At the CRL, however, the CPG acts as a script, almost a recipe to direct the pharmaceutical recovery of soldiers institutionally. Thus, this document is not understood as a list of recommendations that health care workers can refer to in order to supplement and inform specific treatment cases. Instead, at the CRL, the CPG becomes a military protocol—a set of strict and defined rules that *must be followed* word for word and whose disregard can lead to disciplinary and legal punishments. In fact, within the Army, the CPG is not called *la guía* (the guideline) as it is everywhere else, but *el protocolo* (the protocol).

Having a *protocol* was very useful for the major who led the CRL during my fieldwork there because it allowed him to understand all the necessary steps in the medical management of leishmaniasis patients and, thus, the obligations of both soldiers and medical personnel. More importantly, the CPG enabled him to manage the length of each step of the processes. In other words, the major used the CPG as a tool for ensuring that medical procedures and recovery were occurring at an optimal pace. "Here, I use a sentence for those who work for me. I tell people 'It's not important how many people come to the CRL. The important thing is that people are leaving [the facility].' I mean, there really can't be people *mamando gallo* [fooling around], there can't be soldiers who have finished the treatment and are still here without anybody telling them anything." According to the major, "activating the protocol" meant under no circumstances exceeding the treatment and observation times indicated in the CPG. He explained to me that the Army measured his and the CRL's productivity according to the number of patients treated. Thus, a main part of his job was to ensure that no soldier-patient stayed in the facility any longer than indicated by the protocol. As such, within this military clinic, the medical procedures as dictated by the CPG serve as a template for maintaining military discipline among both patients and personnel. This document is the basis for medical and military practices and discourses to come together and produce disciplined patients and medical staff dedicated to the mission of rehabilitating soldiers for their efficient return to war.

However, treating a list of medical recommendations as a set of inflexible rules can be risky. An example of this, which I regularly observed at the CRL, was the medical treatment of soldiers whose lesions had already scarred without any medication or therapy before they arrived at the CRL. Leishmaniasis sometimes heals on its own, so scientists use the terms *self-resolving* or *spontaneous healing* to describe leishmaniasis lesions that heal without any treatment. According to a systematic review of studies that either used placebos or withheld treatment from leishmaniasis patients in the Americas, spontaneous healing occurred in 6 to 26 percent of the patients and varied based on the parasite species (Fernandes Cota et al. 2016). The 2010 version of the CPG used during my fieldwork did not explain how to handle cases that had self-resolved but did emphasize that every patient with a positive diagnosis should receive Glucantime (see MinSalud 2010), and the Army strictly applied this rule to the letter. Thus, Glucantime was in these instances needlessly administered to soldier-patients who had already recovered on their own, with all the bureaucracy, paperwork, costs, pain, and toxicity that this treatment involves.

When I asked CRL physicians why soldier-patients whose lesions had healed after their diagnosis and before they reached the CRL received twenty days of Glucantime treatment like everybody else, the standard answer was that the procedure was necessary to kill the parasites in their bodies. However, it is now widely accepted that while Glucantime therapy does help in the scarring process of the lesions, it does not guarantee the complete elimination of parasites—known as parasitological cure. In fact, the persistence of *Leishmania* parasites in the body despite Glucantime treatment "is the norm rather than the exception" (Martínez-Valencia et al. 2017, 8). Therefore, it seems that there is not much of a difference in the end result between a successful Glucantime treatment and a body capable of defending itself from the *Leishmania* infection. However, there is a significant difference between someone who has undergone Glucantime treatment and someone who has not. Thus, the verbatim interpretation given to the 2010 CPG within the CRL resulted in the unnecessary exposure of many soldiers—perhaps hundreds—to Glucantime's toxic effects over many years. This might be why the 2018 CPG included the following note, highlighted in bold: "If the patient has a confirmed diagnosis and the lesion heals while undergoing pretreatment laboratory testing, and clinical criteria for healing are met at the medical evaluation, NO treatment should be administered, and strict follow-up must be performed" (MinSalud 2018, 12).

During my fieldwork, I noticed that the CRL was probably the only facility where the CPG's written directions were actually carried out. Not even at LERI—the biomedical research institute where I also conducted ethnographic research—are the medical procedures recommended by the CPG followed with such literal rigor. From the viewpoint of EBM advocates who see standards as prescriptive documents delineating how medical decisions *should* be made and how patients *should* be treated, the CRL would be an "ideal" site where the hopes regarding standardized leishmaniasis therapy in Colombia materialize. In this sense, it could be said that the CRL is a unique facility that follows the CPG's recommendations as envisioned by the board of experts who created the document.

The CPG seems to work best within the Army, suggesting that it was designed specifically for the military environment, with its strict authoritarianism and the disciplinary subjection of the soldier and medical staff. Interestingly, unlike the 2010 CPG, the 2018 CPG indicate that this document was created with input not only from scientists and public officers but also people responsible for considering the Army's institutional context and regarding the soldier as the typical leishmaniasis patient. The head of epidemiological surveillance of the Public Force, the head of operational health of the Army, and the vector-borne diseases coordinator of the Army were three of the twenty experts who created the 2018 CPG. Yet this clinical standard is supposed to work for everyone affected by leishmaniasis in Colombia—not only for soldiers. As I have shown, civilian leishmaniasis sufferers in rural and remote areas of Colombia have very different experiences compared to Army personnel. Civilian access to diagnosis and treatment is characterized by (mis)encounters with the state across challenging therapeutic itineraries, full of obstacles and barriers erected on the basis of health and war strategies.

This incongruity was particularly evident in my conversation with Tomás Espitia, a physician with a graduate degree in public health and epidemiology. Tomás is convinced that EBM and standardizing health care are key to making the most effective public policy decisions regarding health. When I met him in 2017, Tomás was working on the CPG update that would be released a year later by MinSalud. Regarding the prospect of implementing this new version in the Army, Tomás said:

> I think that the implementation [of the 2018 CPG] in military environments is even easier, first because the military environment, speaking of the Army,

> as a regime of exception, has different considerations in relation to the provision of services and access to them. Compared to a soldier, it's different, [for example] if a boy from an Indigenous community, with cutaneous leishmaniasis on his little leg, needs to be moved [for him to access health care]. Most likely, the soldier will be evacuated from that area earlier than the child, right? So, I believe that implementation and access may be even more feasible in the case of the military.

It was clear to Tomás that applying the CPG to help civilians affected by the disease would be highly challenging, to say the least. In contrast, the CPG is a perfect fit for the Army, as it seamlessly integrates into the military setting and easily meets the goal of standardizing medical procedures for treating soldiers with leishmaniasis. More importantly, the CPG allows for the creation of an efficient system to administer Glucantime to soldiers, helping them return to their duties on the battlefield as quickly as possible. It also teaches military administrators and health care staff how to manage a disease with which they were completely unfamiliar. In other words, the current CPG emphasizes that its functionality—its capacity to be put into use—is mainly focused on meeting the needs of the military community rather than those of the civilian and rural populations. As Stefan Timmermans and Steven Epstein have written: "Standards are presumed to be in the public interest, but the public to whom standards apply is usually not directly represented in standard creation" (2010, 77). The clinical guidelines created by the Colombian state for treating leishmaniasis patients all over the country does not accurately represent the conditions of the civilian with leishmaniasis, especially when compared to those of the soldier with leishmaniasis.

Stefan Timmermans and Marc Berg (2003) have argued that medical standards are world-making objects, contextually situated, and inherently political. In their words, "Standards are not one uniform thing, with one uniform effect. They help to bring into existence new ideas, entities, values, and even subjects of medicine" (2003, 23). In a military setting, the state's clinical practice standard has become a military protocol enabling the disciplinary control of medical staff and soldier-patients involved in the pharmaceutical treatment of leishmaniasis. By meticulously following every instruction in this document, administrators and health workers at the CRL use the CPG as a script that stipulates the administration of Glucantime injections for the efficient redeployment of soldiers and maintenance of the war machine. The strictness that characterizes how the CPG is used within the Colombian Army highlights the risks of interpreting medical standards as rigid rules instead of recommendations or guidelines. In this case, the inflexible interpretation of the leishmaniasis guidelines resulted in the administration of a highly toxic drug to patients who did not need it. This would indicate that for a medical standard to function ideally, it is necessary for these documents to not only allow but also *promote* freedom in clinical practice and emphasize the centrality of the patient's safety and well-being. Even in a military context, it remains true that "a standard's flexibility is often key to its success" (Timmermans and Epstein 2010, 81).

Additionally, the fact that the CPG's capacity to be put into use can only be guaranteed in a medical-military setting like the CRL raises concerns about its use outside of military contexts. It is doubtful whether standardized health care can be provided for civilian patients with leishmaniasis because of the significant limitations and barriers in accessing quality health care services, diagnosis, treatment, and medical follow-up in rural areas. The expected benefits of standardized medicine are called into question when it cannot be implemented. As in other geographical areas where medical standards must perform under conditions "largely incapable of providing adequate material support for the implementation of EBM" (Geltzer 2009, 526), equitable and war-free access to leishmaniasis therapy is a basic requirement for the standardization of the clinical management of this disease.

WARTIME HEALTH CARE INNOVATIONS

After the daily session of injections at the CRL, the female nursing assistants went to the Healing Room.[16] There, they would take care of groups of two to three soldiers that, in the span of one and a half hours, continuously entered and left the room. Each soldier was asked to expose the part of his body where the leishmaniasis lesion was located. One of the patients, Corporal Nieto, had an ulcer under his left knee on the outside of his leg. Alba, one of the nursing assistants, stripped the bandage and, after carefully rubbing a gauze strip around the ulcer, removed all of the yellowish scabs with a swab. She then used a blade to carefully shave the leg's hairs, which, according to her, were contributing to the infection. She cleaned the area once more, including the hollow and raw section of the lesion. Corporal Nieto writhed in pain, but Alba quickly completed the most painful part of the cleaning. Finally, she applied a topical antibiotic and Crema No. 4 (a diaper cream) around the lesion to keep the skin moist and elastic. She finished by patiently and meticulously covering the sore with gauze and holding it in place with several strips of surgical tape.

Meanwhile, Marisol, another nursing assistant, worked on soldier Herrera's lesion, which was on the back of his ankle. Since his ulcer was very large, extremely infected, and foul smelling, Marisol asked Herrera to stand next to the stretcher, bend his leg, and put his ankle over a plastic bin. As she poured a stream of disinfectant on the ulcer, Herrera's body language expressed agony. Marisol cleaned the lesion thoroughly. Around the ulcer, she applied a white cream she had prepared herself according to a "secret formula" she developed over many years of dealing with a wide variety of leishmaniasis lesions in the Army. In the center of the lesion—the hole—she put unflavored gelatin powder. Marisol and many others explained to me that gelatin's role was the same as that of grated *panela* (unrefined whole cane sugar): *llamar carne* (attract flesh). "As days go by, you begin to see how, thanks to gelatin or *panela*, the hole gets filled with flesh again," she told me. Finally, she covered the ulcer with gauze and told Herrera to see her again in two days. "Marisol has divine hands, that's her reputation here," Herrera told me later.

In addition to these skillful procedures, Alba, Marisol, and the other nursing assistants sometimes injected the lesions with corticosteroids to help lower the inflammation around the edges. They also administered local anesthesia before debridement, a procedure that removes dead, damaged, or infected skin tissue to improve and promote the healing process of the ulcers.

The curative practices performed in the CRL's Healing Room are exclusive to the management of leishmaniasis patients within this military facility. They are not part of the CPG's recommendations and are not commonly used in nonmilitary medical settings. Within the military context, the development and customary use of curative strategies have been crucial in addressing the fact that Glucantime alone is often insufficient to heal an ulcer and form a scar. In the Army, this is especially true for large lesions that result when soldiers with leishmaniasis are not promptly evacuated from the jungle. Servicemen often refer to their ulcers as *monedas* (coins) not only to describe their shape but also because many of their superiors wait for the lesion to reach the size of a 500-peso coin (or a Gatorade cap) to evacuate them. "There are very despotic commanders," soldiers often complained. "They leave you in the area of operations until you have a very big lesion." As a result, it is not uncommon to see ulcers like Herrera's in the CRL. Many of these lesions are concave, circular, and oozing holes in the skin that measure from 4 to 6 centimeters in diameter.

Leishmaniasis lesions may persist despite Glucantime treatment administered according to CPG guidelines. The experiences of soldiers at the CRL confirm that this "therapeutic failure" or "Glucantime resistance," as physicians and scientists call it, is not necessarily due to the drug not being administered according to the CPG's recommendations. Simply put, sometimes Glucantime does not work. Soldiers who do not respond to this drug as expected must undergo additional antileishmanial treatments. Beyond question, without the careful healing work of the CRL nursing assistants, many more soldiers would be classified as therapeutic failures and forced to endure more cycles of therapy. Because of the high level of exposure to all manner of leishmaniasis lesions, CRL medical staff have gained extensive practical knowledge in treating leishmaniasis ulcers that is virtually unique to the CRL. If the state acknowledged the importance of this practical knowledge and applied it to the civilian population, it could reduce treatment failure and the repeated use of harmful drugs among leishmaniasis patients. Moreover, these practices could encourage the urgent adoption of local therapies in Colombia to address the harm caused by the extended and systemic use of Glucantime (Pinto-García 2022, 2025).

Nonetheless, the Army's primary goal in developing these innovative health care practices is not to improve soldiers' health but to promote rapid scarring of their lesions so they can return to battle as soon as possible. Using the same logic, the CRL uses new and exceptional forms of physiotherapy to rehabilitate soldier-patients not from leishmaniasis but from the effects of Glucantime therapy. One of the most common reasons to suspend treatment—significantly delaying the soldier's discharge—is that the injections can damage the muscles of the buttocks and cause abscesses to form. This is especially frequent and painful in soldier-patients with larger buttocks who tend to retain more of the injected liquid. During my fieldwork, Milena Rojas, a civilian physiotherapist, was in charge of daily massaging and applying heat and cold therapy to soldiers to reduce swelling and the accumulation of Glucantime in the buttock muscle fibers. In the more chronic cases, she also used electrotherapy and ultrasound. When I asked about how this practice began, Milena replied as follows:

> In the past, an officer in charge of the CRL realized that the physiotherapy service was needed given all the adverse events they had. There were many patients [whose Glucantime treatments] were suspended because of [problems with] their buttocks. As a result, the soldiers' stay [in the CRL] was much longer. This was very problematic for the battalions because very large groups could arrive—20 soldiers, 15 soldiers could arrive from a single battalion. Then, the battalion was left without people and this was a problem for the commanders. As a result, [the administration of the CRL] realized that physiotherapy was needed as part of the process.

Milena also explained to me that, in her work outside the Army, she had never met patients whose buttocks were affected to the same extent as those undergoing Glucantime treatment. "Not even with other kinds of injections?" I asked. "No, it's just supremely rare. The doses [of Glucantime] are very high and, apart from that, they are daily, so here one sees buttocks *vueltos nada* [badly hurt]. It is a supremely strong medicine, and it damages the muscle fibers. That's what produces abscesses. It damages the fibers, it damages the skin, it damages everything. That can even have long-term consequences, which also depends a lot on the size of the buttocks."

The case of soldier Cubides is illustrative in this regard. During an injection session, nursing assistant Camila was preparing to inject 10 ml of Glucantime into the buttocks of Cubides, one of the heaviest soldier-patients at the CRL. But she could not complete the task. During the previous days of treatment, the medicine had accumulated in the muscle fibers, causing firm and painful abscesses on both sides. "Sometimes the liquid does not get into the gluteus anymore; those *muchachos* [young men] cannot even sit," Camila told me later. With the help of a general practitioner, Camila used four 5-ml syringes to drain 20 ml of blood, pus, and accumulated Glucantime from Cubides's buttocks. After that impressive and tense procedure, which got the attention of everyone in the Injection Room, Cubides stood up, looking relieved. In the days to come, I would see him visiting the Physiotherapy Room every day until his treatment could resume.

Although Milena believes that physical therapy is absolutely necessary for soldiers to be able to endure Glucantime injections, she also thinks that leishmaniasis patients should receive physical therapy sessions after the treatment. This, however, does not happen in the Army, let alone outside of it. In her opinion, this would greatly help people undergoing such an intense treatment to regain some weight and muscle mass without excessively straining the heart, which is heavily impacted by Glucantime. In the case of soldiers, she says, this would promote better physical and emotional conditions before returning them to their military work. In Milena's view, her profession was well positioned to do this because

> physiotherapy is a way of approaching a patient, a human being, not in the traditional way, as a physician does, using medicines only. I like physiotherapy because you really interact with the person—you handle not just bodies, but souls, everything. You handle a lot of emotions. More than manipulating a body, one handles what we call corporeality. Then, we deal with emotions, we deal with the relationship with other people. And all that helps soldiers to relieve pain. So you may not have done much to him, but you told him a joke and made him feel good. The next day they come here to thank you that their buttocks are not hurting anymore. So it's nice to get them out of their routine and their military role.

Despite the importance of physiotherapy for soldiers undergoing leishmaniasis treatment, at the end of my fieldwork at the CRL, the DISAN had decided that it would not rehire a CRL physiotherapist due to budget cuts. Soldiers who needed this service would have to go to the dispensary of the Silva Plazas Battalion and request an appointment to receive physiotherapy sessions. This, of course, was a major setback for soldiers' physical and emotional recovery process.

The curative practices and physiotherapy sessions provided to soldiers at the CRL are not included in the CPG. Although CRL medical staff strictly follow the CPG recommendations, they also work *beyond* it by implementing new practices that help soldiers heal, recover from the harmful effects of Glucantime, and return to the area of operations more quickly. Although "standards promise to provide the optimal technical solution for particular problems" (Timmermans and Epstein 2010, 73–74), the military environment in which the leishmaniasis CPG is embedded demands much more from medical practitioners. If it weren't for the supplementary work carried out by CRL health personnel, the CPG would fall short in healing soldier-patients with leishmaniasis. These efforts ensure that the standards do not fail to deliver the promised results and protect this document's usefulness and credibility.

Since the mid-2000s, the extensive use of antileishmanial drugs has become crucial in maximizing the labor capacity of soldiers with the disease. In addition to using Glucantime to address the shortage of soldiers, the Army adopted the MinSalud CPG and turned it into a military protocol that produces disciplined patients and medical personnel, engaged in the mission of returning soldiers to the area of operations as quickly and efficiently as possible. With the same objective, the Army also established unparalleled facilities and developed innovative health procedures such as curative practices and physiotherapy. Thus, the mutual reinforcement of war and technoscience in the Army led to an accelerated system of treating leishmaniasis to speed up the scarring process and send soldiers back to the forest to fight the war against guerrillas and other armed actors in contemporary Colombia.

4
Glucantime and the Politics of Cure

The day I started my ethnographic research at the CRL, I witnessed a scene that would be repeated every morning of my fieldwork (fig. 4.1). Fifteen or so men gathered in front of the central building, roaming around and rubbing their buttocks with gestures of discomfort and pain. Each had just received two injections of Glucantime. Some of the men had gauze bandages that covered leishmaniasis ulcers on the face, scalp, neck, or hands. Others had their lesions hidden under the mandatory "sick-men uniform"—a dark blue sweatshirt with red seams and the Colombian Army insignia embroidered in red. They looked ill, weak, vulnerable, and childlike—quite the opposite of the image of strong and tough men usually associated with the military.

One of these sick soldiers was Pacheco. When we met, he had spent twelve of his thirty-two years of life in the Army and was one of the very few leishmaniasis patients in the CRL who was older than thirty. Pacheco was born in the south of the *departamento* of Bolívar, in a town historically devastated by violence. Although he only studied until the third grade of primary school, his arithmetic skills were notorious among the petty gambling circle that operated in the lower part of the central bunkbed in one of the two CRL dormitories (fig. 4.2). At eleven, Pacheco began working in clandestine coca plantations as a *raspachín* (coca harvester), often moving from place to place throughout rural Colombia in search of coca crops ready to be stripped of their leaves. While in the coca business, Pacheco made about two million pesos a month (about 761 USD in 2004), significantly more than what he was making as a professional soldier (about 316 USD in 2016). He used to spend that money mostly on cockfight bets, alcohol, and sex workers. That was his life until the age of twenty.

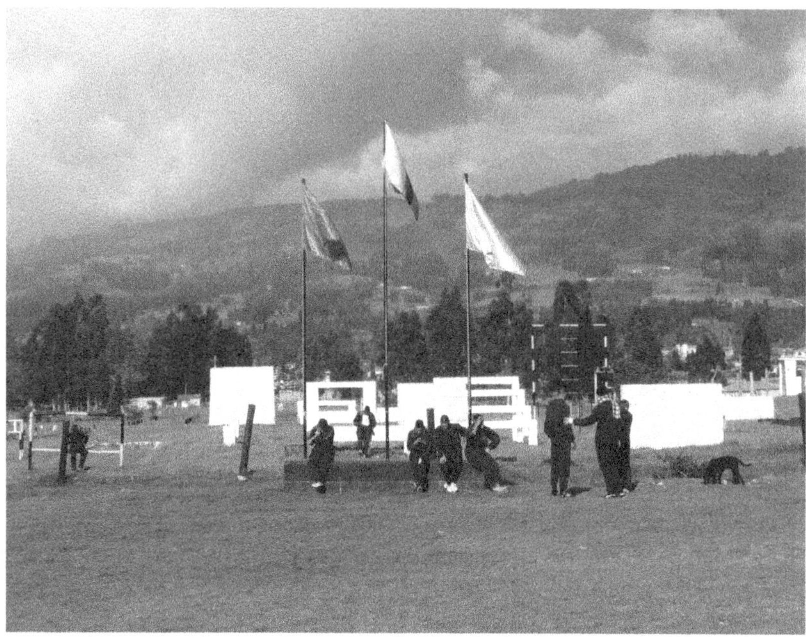

FIGURE 4.1. Soldiers with leishmaniasis, minutes after being injected with Glucantime at the CRL. Photo by Lina Pinto-García.

Tired of that nomadic routine, Pacheco decided to join the Army. I asked him if he had not contemplated other options. "Joining guerrilla or paramilitary groups," he replied. Those were the only three alternatives this young rural man, with little education, had envisaged for himself. Despite the life-threatening risks and mistreatments associated with soldiering in Colombia, many young people from marginalized sectors of society consider the Army to be an appealing option. Joining the Army ensures job security, provides the peace of mind of having a legal occupation, prevents recruitment by guerrilla and paramilitary groups, and offers the possibility of retiring at an early age—if you manage to stay alive long enough. Moreover, the Army allows recruits to build family-like bonds with other soldiers and experience a deeply felt camaraderie and sense of belonging that is rarely found outside the military (Carmona Lozano 2016; Forero Ángel 2017). Thus, Pacheco's decision to join the Army was not surprising—rather, it was a common solution to the structural inequities and lack of opportunities that many young people in Colombia face, especially in rural areas.

Pacheco approached the closest battalion but was denied admission because of health problems with his teeth and spine. Refusing to take no for an answer and with less than 50,000 pesos (about 19 USD in 2004) in his pocket,

Pacheco gathered a group of sixteen young men, convinced them to join the Army, and introduced them to a subofficer. As a reward for supplying the Army with so many new recruits, Pacheco was drafted as well. He served in the military for two years as a regular soldier but, once he regained civilian status, he eventually started to miss military life. "Something about the Army has to appeal to you for you to stay here," he said apologetically. To qualify for admission despite his health issues, he had to bribe the Army officials in charge of processing his enrollment.

After completing the four months of training required to become a professional soldier, Pacheco spent most of his time patrolling rural areas in southern Colombia. It was there that, in 2008, he became infected with *Leishmania* parasites for the first time. When the troop commander finally gave the order to evacuate him from the area of operations, the ulcer was already quite large and, therefore, Glucantime therapy did not heal it. As a result, Pacheco received another complete cycle—another twenty days—of Glucantime. This time, the lesion healed. However, ten days after returning to his military unit, Pacheco had to go back into the jungle, and he eventually developed leishmaniasis lesions on other areas of his body. Once again, he was given Glucantime. He returned to the area of operations, but the first lesion

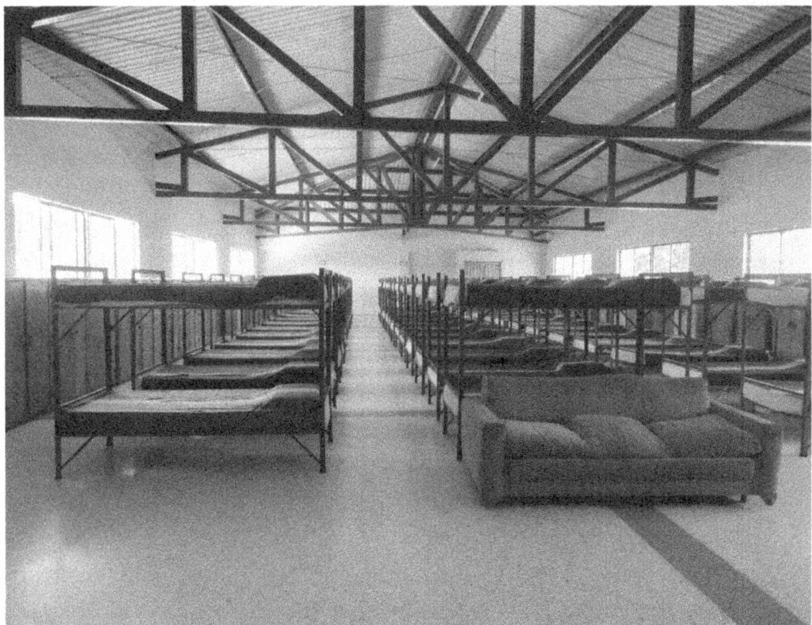

FIGURE 4.2. One of the two CRL dormitories. Photo by Lina Pinto-García.

had reopened. As it was an "old" lesion, Pacheco was sent to the BASAN in Bogotá, to be treated with pentamidine, a second-line leishmaniasis drug that is similarly toxic to Glucantime. This decision to administer pentamidine is based on the assumption that leishmaniasis lesions that appear on different parts of the body and at different times are not caused by the same *Leishmania* infection. However, as I explained in the previous chapter, it is well accepted that Glucantime treatment does not guarantee the complete elimination of parasites in the body. Thus, establishing a clinical difference between the reactivation of an "old" lesion and the manifestation of a "new" infection is misleading. Therefore, it is possible that Pacheco's second encounter with leishmaniasis was caused by the same *Leishmania* parasites that were already in his body from the first infection. Moreover, Glucantime might not work a second time if it did not work previously, as in Pacheco's case. It is logical to assume that if Glucantime did not cause scarring in the past, it might be unable to do so in the future. This consideration has often been disregarded by military medicine in Colombia.

After the pentamidine treatment, Pacheco returned to work. However, after several months, leishmaniasis lesions reappeared—this time on his face. By the time I met Pacheco at the CRL in 2016, he was recovering from his fifth antileishmanial treatment in a span of less than ten years—four times with Glucantime and once with pentamidine. When I asked for his thoughts on the long-term effects of these medications on his body, he said:

> I liked to jog a lot. Now, I can no longer stand a physical test of two miles, I can't stand it. Halfway through it . . . I have to walk because I feel breathless. . . . In the area of operations, when I'm walking, it's the same. If I carry a lot of weight, and I am, say, going up a slope or a hill, I have to take several breaks because I just can't do it all at once as I used to. . . . Not anymore. Now I need several breaks of one, two, three minutes before I can resume walking.

Worried and still in pain from the injections and toxic effects of Glucantime, Pacheco told me that after his discharge from the CRL, he wanted to pay for several diagnostic tests to determine the condition of his heart, liver, pancreas, and kidneys after so many antileishmanial treatments. He also wanted to understand why he had not been able to have children, a problem he suspected was related to the medications used to treat leishmaniasis.[1] "Before the treatment, did the medical personnel mention to you what the possible consequences of the drug were?" I asked. Pacheco replied: "No, here they only tell you that you can't drink alcohol, that you can't smoke, that you can't drink black beverages [e.g., Coca-Cola and black coffee]. But they never go into detail about issues related to long-term reactions to the drug."

Up to this point, the reader may have mistakenly believed that, compared to the rest of the population, Army soldiers are the only leishmaniasis patients in Colombia whose treatment and recovery are fairly straightforward. After all, servicemen who become infected with *Leishmania* in the "heroic act" of fighting the state enemies are guaranteed state protection in terms of access to pharmaceutical treatment and medically supervised recovery. However, as I have previously shown, the problem posed by the *maraña* formed by leishmaniasis and the armed conflict goes beyond questions of inclusion regarding access to the necessary medicines. The soldier's experience with leishmaniasis, characterized by easy access to Glucantime and its harmful effects, is quite revealing in this context. In this chapter, I show how violence is inflicted not only on rural residents who are denied access to Glucantime but also on Army soldiers when the only alternative that biomedicine and public health choose to offer is highly toxic drugs to treat a disease that is not even fatal.

Here, I examine a crucial thread holding the *maraña* together: the soldier's subjective experience with leishmaniasis and the gradual erosion of his body as a result of antileishmanial drugs whose long-term effects are poorly researched. Thousands of Army members in Colombia—young men from low-income and commonly rural families who usually join the Army out of obligation or necessity—have endured at least one cycle of physical intoxication and deterioration due to the relatively minor and non-life-threatening disease of leishmaniasis. Through their stories, I highlight the drama that this illness and its treatment signify for a large sector of the Colombian population who, while serving and working for the Army, have endured the known and unknown consequences of antileishmanial drugs throughout many years of armed conflict. Their experiences show that the pharmaceuticalization of war results in violence not only by excluding the nonmilitary population from accessing medication but also by causing excessive drug use among military personnel. I discuss the rarely mentioned consequences of war caused by the slow destruction of marginalized individuals through pharmacological treatments. These cases remind us that within every pharmaceutical "is a version of the *pharmakon* analyzed by Jacques Derrida—a thing that is both cure and poison" (Greene and Sismondo 2015, 1). The experience of soldiers with leishmaniasis makes us question the extent to which drugs are actually cures in a war context. We must also ask whether the acceptable limits of such a cure moves toward the domain of poison when it comes to winning a war that demands the sacrifice of bodies considered disposable.

Curing Disposable Bodies

In his study of the rollout of ART in Brazil, João Biehl (2007) acknowledges how these treatments improve the morbidity and mortality rates among people infected with HIV. However, his work warns against reducing public health management of a disease to the simple dispensation of "magic bullet" pharmaceutical treatments, as this approach ignores social, economic, and political factors and can perpetuate inequality. As such, the notion of the *pharmaceuticalization of public health* assumes an ambivalent position toward drugs—pharmaceuticals can save lives and improve disease outcomes, but they can also obscure social complexities and ignore the fundamental causes of health issues.

In a similar vein, Stefan Ecks (2005) has argued that biomedical discourses tend to use the term *marginalized* for people with no access to pharmaceutical products. He coined the phrase *pharmaceutical citizenship* to explain how pharmaceuticals often constitute "a promise of demarginalization" in contexts where these technologies are not equally available to everyone (2005, 241). Under these circumstances, providing medications to treat underserved people is presented as the most effective way to overcome social marginalization and reintegrate people into society (2005). Although Ecks is a critical of pharmaceuticals, he stresses the importance of approaching health care in a way that "neither reduces it to the proper distribution of medicines, nor simply rejects medicines as fetishized commodities" (2005, 245).

Similarly, Tom Widger suggests that ambivalence provides a valuable opportunity to reflect on and assess "magic bullet" global health interventions without completely dismissing them. He proposes that we "interrogate the social and political implications of the ambivalence they generate" (2018, 407). Murguía et al. (2016) note that this ambivalence is especially necessary in Latin America, where pharmaceuticals are commonly overprescribed and used excessively, while numerous people die from diseases that can be prevented or cured with proper medication. Therefore, demanding equal access to drugs for all is crucial; however, it is also vital to emphasize that solving public health problems should not rely solely on medication. Moreover, the case of Colombian leishmaniasis and the Glucantime-centered approach to controlling it demonstrates the importance of not accepting the first drug that seems promising for treatment. Although this approach may seem indecisive and contradictory, it is necessary to demand better access to antileishmanial drugs for all while also warning against the indiscriminate use of pharmaceutical solutions and their unequal effects on marginalized groups such as those young men who are more likely to join the Colombian Army than their fellow citizens. Their case highlights the importance of understanding the impact of pharmaceuticalized models of public health on both the excluded and included groups.

Disability studies are helpful when examining the politics of cure in the drug-centered management of leishmaniasis in Colombia's military. Eli Clare's work (2017) is particularly valuable for exploring the ambivalent nature of medical treatments among disabled people. Clare illuminates and problematizes the experiential, embodied, and subjective aspects of the pharmaceuticalization of public health that I explore here. He argues that ableism often takes the form of the assumption that disabilities are body-mind defects that require medical treatment to be prevented and eradicated. This *ideology of cure*, as Clare calls it, promises that disabled people will not only be cured but that all manner of disabilities will eventually disappear. He responds to this with a vehement anticure politics emphasizing that disability does not equate to damage, lack of health, or defect. What disabled people need, he argues, is not a cure but "civil rights, equal access, gainful employment, the opportunity to live independently, good and respectful healthcare, [and] unsegregated education" (Eli Clare, as quoted by Clare 2017, 60). Yet he does not reject cure altogether. Aware that some disabled people experience physical and psychological burdens that no amount of social justice can ease, Clare maintains that cures are necessary as long as they are not intended to eradicate people. "Holding it all—sickness and human vulnerability, health and disability, the need for and the rejection of cure—is . . . necessary" (Clare 2017, 62).

Soldiers with leishmaniasis are regarded as defective tools who need pharmaceutical treatment to return to the work of war. However, as soon as they reject treatment or they can no longer perform their work, they are expelled from the Army, losing their status as "privileged" pharmaceutical citizens. Instead of ensuring a healthy and meaningful life for these men beyond their role as soldiers, pharmaceutical regimes of war focus on treating them only until they are no longer useful to the Army. In this case, the ideology of cure aims to repair bodies as much as possible for use in war and eliminate them if they can no longer serve war's objectives. While the soldier's ability to fight is repaired in the short term, the human being is rendered incapable in the long run. Jasbir K. Puar calls this the *biopolitics of debilitation*—"the slow wearing down of populations instead of the event of becoming disabled" (Puar 2017, xiv). Although debilitation caused by Glucantime is considered to be a normal and expected consequence of being a soldier, the use of this drug is in fact a pharmaceutical way of extracting value "from populations that would otherwise be disposable" (Puar 2017, xviii). In other words, the medical treatment of soldiers with leishmaniasis exemplifies the state-sanctioned violence—justified in the protectionist terms of health care—that Puar (2017) calls *the right to maim*. The state claims the right to harm soldiers not only through the direct violence of war but also through medical treatment for a disease they contract while fighting that war. Expanding on Puar's work, I observe a maiming system in action, a "will not let die" mindset applied to men whose bodies are needed to fight a war but whose debilitation is not necessarily a loss but an "externality" of the armed conflict. It is undeniable that Glucantime is effective in treating leishmaniasis lesions,[2] but the experience of Colombian soldiers highlights the harmful effects of this highly toxic approach to managing a mostly benign skin disease. Although some armed nonstate actors and civilians may have access to the same treatment as soldiers, the repeated administration of antileishmanial drugs in the military (which may include up to six treatments!) is a very specific and extreme case. Soldiers treated in this manner serve as an extreme example of what occurs in nonmilitary populations undergoing systemic treatment with Glucantime. Their experiences underscore the dangers of a public health policy that should be critically evaluated and radically changed as a matter of urgency.

As Clare makes clear, cure as ideology disregards the side effects of the cure and considers them preferable to the condition of disability because this ideology's purpose is to eliminate disability at any cost. While some medical treatments work most of the time for most people, others "offer glimmers of possibility but present high risks or ambiguous outcomes" (Clare 2017, 76). In those cases, "we—the consumers, clients or patients—are often blamed, either subtly or blatantly, for these failures. We didn't try hard enough. We were lazy. We were drug resistant. We were noncompliant. . . . Somehow, amidst it all, the very notion of cure remains undisputed" (2017, 77). Challenging this aspect of the ideology of cure means resisting the assumption that all pharmaceuticals are better than the disease itself or that pharmaceuticals are inherently good. It also forces us to critically examine the poisonous properties of drugs and the adoption of pharmaceuticals as a one-size-fits-all approach that becomes naturalized despite the serious problems it can present.

To evaluate the historical use of Glucantime in Colombia, we must consider the consequences of the pharmaceuticalization of public health when it is found *enmarañado* with war-based citizenship systems and ideologies of cure. This approach demands an examination of how bodies that are governed by this ideology experience antileishmanial treatment. Furthermore, it raises the question of whether national regulations to control leishmaniasis would prioritize such a harmful drug if this disease were affecting a different social group. In the following sections, I focus on the physical legacies of

Glucantime in lower-ranking military groups, which the state and Colombian society exploit to wage a war that pits the poor against the poor.

A Sick Soldier Is a Bad Soldier

At the CRL, I witnessed how Glucantime was injected into dozens of soldiers with leishmaniasis every day. Soldiers commonly used the word *veneno* (poison) to refer to this drug. Many of these young men suffered greatly when their ulcers were not healing or when the drug made them feel so sick and miserable they thought they were dying. Most of them, however, avoided showing their distress because the typical response they received sought to undermine their suffering and challenge their masculinity. *No venda lástima* (don't sell pity) was the sentence their peers and CRL staff repeatedly used. Some soldiers disliked the forceful approach of Glucantime therapy and would have preferred to be treated with *rezos* (prayers) and plant-based remedies often found in rural areas (see Pinto-García 2025). I heard some of them express deep fear of the disease mostly because they had seen others return from their treatment in such bad shape that they had to *pedir la baja* (retire from the Army) and go back to "being nothing, not even a soldier," as one of them told me.

Suspicion and antipathy characterized most of the interactions between a soldier-patient and the CRL staff. The latter often thought that the soldier was somehow undermining his recovery, not making an effort, or taking the responsibility to heal and recover. Many soldiers were made to feel guilty, proving that "militaries think soldiers are never quite up to the tasks at hand and are liable to fail at any moment" (Bickford 2020, 1). A soldier's alleged lack of cooperation was often referenced in terms of immoral behavior through humiliating comments about his assumed uncontrolled sexuality—unable to stop masturbating or looking for sex workers—and his decadent and inevitable tendency toward drug and alcohol consumption. Moreover, when ulcers persisted despite treatment, the blame was usually placed on the soldier's (generally presumed) objectionable behavior rather than on Glucantime's deficiencies. As Eli Clare (2017) rightly points out, when a drug does not work well, it is the patients who are somehow responsible, not the ideology that considers cures to be unquestionably beneficial.

"A sick soldier is a bad soldier," Velandia told me. For him, a professional soldier with eleven years of Army experience, that is the way servicemen with leishmaniasis are usually regarded by commanders, officers, and military doctors. In the opinion of a military physician, "Every man with leishmaniasis is a man who is not in the place where he should be—in his combat workplace, in the battalion fulfilling a certain function." Perhaps for that reason, commanders and medical personnel often see leishmaniasis as an illness that soldiers bring upon themselves, a disciplinary failure, a sign of weakness, or evidence for deceptive behavior. The assumption seemed to be that *all* soldiers were always mischievously and actively trying to get bitten by sandflies so they could have several months of rest at the CRL and avoid returning to work.

When I asked servicemen and CRL staff members if they believed the disease carried a stigma, instead of referring to "the guerrilla disease," many replied: "Yes, the stigma of being a bad soldier." Kenneth MacLeish has documented a similar way of blaming US soldiers for their illnesses and health problems: "Claiming to suffer from pain and discomfort typically earns a soldier little more than the suspicion of his commanders, fellows, and doctors" (2013, 104). The Colombian Army's discriminatory way of understanding leishmaniasis has been particularly evident in the internal calls for Special Forces training opportunities. These are six-month courses where professional soldiers learn to perform complex air, land, and water operations with the highest level of military training (Ejército Nacional 2016). According to Velandia, the calls indicate that only those professional soldiers "with three to five years of military experience, no legal or health problems, and who have never had leishmaniasis are eligible. But how many professional soldiers with that experience have not had the disease? My estimate is less than 20 percent. Many good soldiers miss out on opportunities because of having had leishmaniasis. There are good soldiers who have had leishmaniasis; they deserve to be sent to that training, to get some fresh air, to gain knowledge that could help them request a transfer." But they cannot advance because their medical record is stained by leishmaniasis, a disease they acquire while being soldiers.

During my field research, I heard about soldiers using leishmaniasis as a way to resist and cope with the challenges of military life. Immersed in the daily life of combat, exhausted from months in the jungle, unable to communicate with their families, or simply fed up with war, some soldiers bared their torsos and rolled up their trousers at twilight to get bitten by sandflies. I was also told about soldiers who "saved the lesion for Christmas," meaning they would put off telling their commanders about their ulcers so their treatments would be delayed until a special time of the year when they hoped to be with, near, or at least in phone contact with their families. I met soldiers who wanted to time their scarring period so that their time at the CRL and their leave would align. In this way, they could prolong their time away from the tropical forest as much as possible. I also heard that leishmaniasis treatment could be a lucky misfortune because it kept some soldiers away from combat or ambushes that they might not have survived. These practices are small in scale but crucial to subverting the daily violence soldiers experience on a micro and macro level. Manuel Tironi (2018) calls such acts *hypo-interventions*—forms of intimate activism. They are also mundane and unspectacular responses to pharmaceutical harm that—like toxicity amid late industrial developmentalism—is diffuse, unseen, gradual, and slow, affecting some bodies and not others under specific modes of wartime injustice and sacrifice (Liboiron, Tironi, and Calvillo 2018).

The violence experienced by young soldiers does not end when they leave their area of operations. It goes on in medical and clinical settings when they are treated as being responsible for leishmaniasis and blamed when the treatment does not work. This process of subjectification requires not only the symbolic violence expressed through the constant denigration of soldiers; it also demands that they remain unaware of the bodily and institutional implications of leishmaniasis and its pharmaceutical therapy, as I describe below.

Curing with Pharmaceuticals Requires a Dose of Ignorance

In the CRL, I had several opportunities to witness the exchange between a nurse and a soldier that always preceded the signing of an informed consent form before the Glucantime treatment started. As Pacheco had told me, this discussion focused on telling soldiers that feeling sick because of Glucantime was completely normal and letting them know about the things they were *not* allowed to do: drinking black beverages such as Coca-Cola or *tinto* (black coffee),[3] drinking alcohol, doing cardiovascular activities,[4] taking vitamins,[5] having sex,[6] or impregnating a woman within three months after the treatment. Soldiers were also warned that failure to comply with military discipline, medical procedures, or scheduled medical appointments would be understood as an "abandonment of treatment." In such a case, they were told that they would not be able to request further medical attention from the Army.

This preconsent briefing, however, never included information about leishmaniasis, Glucantime's harmful effects, or the financial compensations to which military members were entitled due to scarring and aftereffects of the treatment. For example, Pacheco found out about his right to financial compensation for his leishmaniasis scars because he befriended one of the CRL military nurses who shared that information with him. Otherwise, like many other soldiers, he might never have known that he could initiate a medical-administrative procedure to receive financial compensation.

The *junta médica* is a military-occupational medical board made up of three military doctors who evaluate Army members' acquired disabilities and medically diagnosed conditions. Its role is to determine whether a person has a disease that the Army considers occupational. This board is also responsible for quantifying the reduction in a soldier's ability to work and deciding whether they are still *apto* (fit) to stay in the Army, if they should be relocated, and if they deserve financial compensation.[7] In the case of leishmaniasis, the *junta médica* determines the economic compensation soldiers receive for both the scarring and the conditions caused by the treatment (heart, liver, kidney, or infertility problems); however, these must be supported by medical exams and diagnostic tests.[8]

I was often present at the medical consultations that soldiers had to attend before, during, and after their Glucantime treatment at the CRL. At one of them, a professional soldier asked the doctor about the *junta médica*. He had been diagnosed with and treated for leishmaniasis once before, so he wanted to know if he should ask the board to review his case. "The Army only pays once for any given pathology," the doctor said. In other words, soldiers are only compensated once for leishmaniasis scars and treatment aftereffects. If he had asked for a *junta médica* review at that point, having undergone "only" two Glucantime treatments, he would have used up his only chance to receive compensation. The doctor went on to explain that because he was going to be sent back to the jungle, he should wait for his fifth antileishmanial treatment. Only then could he ask to be relocated to a different location, possibly in a colder area where there was no chance of getting leishmaniasis again. Thus, the doctor recommended that he wait until his fifth treatment to request an evaluation by the *junta médica*. At that point, the medical board would probably decide to compensate him for *all* of his scars and side effects from *all five* Glucantime treatments. *Véalo como un ahorro* (look at it as savings), the doctor harshly concluded.

During their time in the CRL, soldiers were required to attend several talks on health issues. However, these sessions never mentioned leishmaniasis and were not safe spaces for soldiers to resolve their many concerns about the disease and treatment—concerns they often shared with me in private conversations. For example, they sometimes did not understand how leishmaniasis was transmitted. Soldiers often compared their experiences using the limited biomedical knowledge they had acquired through hearsay. For instance, based on their experience with tick bites, contusions, and wounds that developed into sores, later diagnosed as leishmaniasis, many doubted that it was sandflies that transmitted the disease.

Despite their limited and casually acquired knowledge, servicemen wanted to learn more. They wished to compare their experiences against a fuller picture of biomedical knowledge, verify if their experiences aligned with the claims of scientists and doctors, fill the gaps in their knowledge, and find answers to their many questions. However, opportunities to do these things were systematically denied. For instance, in a talk about sexually transmitted diseases (STDs), a CRL nurse gave a one-hour presentation on syphilis, herpes, papilloma, condyloma, gonorrhea, and HIV/AIDS. Not a word was said about leishmaniasis. When the nurse asked for questions, none of the soldier-patients inquired about STDs. Instead, they asked about the subject that concerned them bodily, emotionally, and intellectually: leishmaniasis. The nurse quickly answered a few questions and called it a day.

Soldiers are kept unaware of the therapeutic details of the disease to make them more likely to accept taking Glucantime despite its harmful effects. This suggests that increased knowledge among soldier-patients about leishmaniasis, antileishmanial treatments, and their rights could disrupt the military's management of the disease. Because the government or military leaders are responsible for wounded and sick soldiers, "military strategists have incentives to deny, underestimate or hide the wounded" (Enloe 2023, 84). Keeping soldiers uninformed saves money and normalizes the risks of leishmaniasis and its treatment within the military. In this way, leishmaniasis stays out of public view and is regarded as an occupational disease that does not deserve attention or wider discussion.

Curable as Long as Usable

A subofficer named Cruz told me that despite receiving Glucantime only once, the medication had caused permanent physical damage. Before treatment, he weighed 72 kg and, like most people, gained weight when he ate a lot or did little physical activity. But when he finished the treatment, his weight was 64 kg. "I've eaten, taken vitamins, purged, taken Ensure, but I've never been able to gain the weight back. At most, I've gone up to 65 kg, but never above that." Since receiving Glucantime, Cruz became extremely thin. The cumulative toxic effects of this and other antileishmanial medications on soldiers like Cruz and Pacheco are incalculable.

While Pacheco was at the BASAN receiving pentamidine to treat his fourth episode of leishmaniasis, two soldiers passed away. One of them died in the hospital, several minutes after an injection of amphotericin B—a third-choice drug for leishmaniasis. The second man, who had been assigned Pacheco's top bunk, died during his treatment with pentamidine. Pacheco described these tragic events to me as follows: "During the whole day, he had a fever and was not feeling good. At night, when we had to stand in formation, we called him, and he said 'No, I'm not going, I've got a lot of fever, and I can't go.' At morning reveille, the time to get up, the guy was already dead. Who knows how many hours he had been like that."

While the exact number of military (and civilian) deaths caused by Glucantime, pentamidine, or other antileishmanial drugs remains unreported, a 2012 journal article references twelve fatalities related to Glucantime use that were documented by the Army, "which is unacceptable for a form of the disease that is not fatal" (López et al. 2012, 5). Leishmaniasis researchers and medical professionals in the military admitted to me that there had been more than several deaths caused by Glucantime and other antileishmanial pharmaceuticals in the Army (see also *El Tiempo* 2007). These soldiers did not die in combat—the kind of death that war deems acceptable. These are the kind of deaths that, even in war, are not supposed to happen. As a military doctor told me: "These are losses that were not necessary." The deaths of soldiers caused by antileishmanial drugs show that, during war, health care treatments and cures can be fatal to those whose lives are considered expendable.

In this chapter, I have discussed the experiences of soldiers with leishmaniasis and the impact and consequences of contracting *Leishmania* parasites while serving in the Colombian Army. In particular, I have observed the gradual weakening of the soldier's body under Glucantime treatment and the exposure to the harmful effects of antimony-based drugs during not just one but several episodes of leishmaniasis. I have shown that, after being pharmaceutically recycled, the soldier's body gradually deteriorates until it is disposable. Through this damaging process, war is not confined to the battlefield of the jungle but extends from the emblematic space of the Colombian armed conflict to clinical settings, with the crucial participation of biomedical knowledge, pharmaceuticals, health care practices, and public health regulations.

Such harmful treatment is allowed to continue when soldiers are not informed about the disease, the treatment, and the financial compensation to which they are entitled. In addition to subjecting soldier-patients to various forms of symbolic violence, I have shown how processes of pharmaceuticalization also require deliberately administered doses of ignorance so that these treatments are accepted as the only solution to a problem by both the patient and society.

The pharmaceuticalization of war does not harm soldiers through a lack of Glucantime but rather through an *excess* of this and other antileishmanial drugs. The exorbitant use of these medicines in the Army underscores that the *enmarañamiento* of leishmaniasis and war is not just a problem of unequal access to pharmacological solutions. It suggests that this entanglement is not solved simply by removing the access barriers around Glucantime.

Acknowledging the suffering of soldiers with leishmaniasis involves addressing the numerous ways their rights are violated during their illness, especially considering the structural conditions that lead them to participate in war and contract the disease.

In a similar vein, throughout several decades of armed conflict in Colombia, there is no documentation exposing the limits of pharmaceuticals such as Glucantime. We do not know what happens to the body after going through so many cycles of such a harmful treatment. We do not know why a soldier never regains his former weight, physical condition, or ability to reproduce even after a single treatment. We do not know the effects of Glucantime ten, twenty, or thirty years after receiving it. In fact, we have no answer to a number of questions posed by thousands of soldiers with leishmaniasis—the *leishmaníacos*, as they sometimes like to call themselves.[9]

Although it is rare for people outside the Army to undergo multiple antileishmanial treatments, it is a frequent occurrence in the Army (*El Tiempo* 2007a; Correa-Cárdenas et al. 2020). In a country where the armed conflict is part of everyday life, we cannot keep ignoring the thousands of soldiers and ex-soldiers who have gone through repetitive cycles of toxic physical side effects due to leishmaniasis treatment.[10] Yet the only therapy that biomedicine and public health systems choose to offer to control this nonfatal disease is a scarring poison that might lead to deadly outcomes. Many choose to leave the Army not because of the fighting but because they cannot stand another leishmaniasis treatment. All this shows in a brutal way that "the restoration of health arrives in many slippery guises." Cures sometimes "result in benefit, but they can also cause individual death and the diminishment of whole groups of people" (Clare 2017, 28).

5

Pacified Scientific Accounts on Leishmaniasis

Colombia has one of the highest incidences of cutaneous leishmaniasis worldwide, but the exact number of cases each year is difficult to determine due to the country's widespread underreporting. According to a study led by the World Health Organization (WHO) aimed to account for underreporting, the actual number of annual cases was estimated to be between 48,000 and 80,100 (Alvar et al. 2012). Despite these estimates, leishmaniasis is far from the most prevalent vector-borne disease in Colombia, and it does not cause the most serious symptoms. Between 1990 and 2016, the state recorded a total of 5,360,134 cases of vector-borne diseases. Of this number, 54.7 percent were attributed to malaria and 24.9 percent to dengue, two diseases that, unlike cutaneous leishmaniasis, can be fatal. Thus, malaria and dengue accounted for 80 percent of the cumulative burden of vector-borne diseases in that period (Padilla et al. 2017). Even so, leishmaniasis is one of the most-researched health conditions in Colombia.

A 2009 study on health research shows that since 1970, research on infectious diseases have received the most substantial financial support from Colciencias, the state agency in charge of funding academic research in Colombia (Jaramillo et al. 2009).[1] Among these diseases, leishmaniasis has consistently ranked in one of the top two positions since 1990, which is reflected in both the number of projects funded and the amounts of funding allocated to them. In other words, leishmaniasis has occupied a prominent position in Colombia's health research agenda, and biomedical research groups working on this disease have benefited from generous financial support compared to other diseases and health concerns. Similarly, in the last four decades, scientific groups dedicated to the biomedical study of leishmaniasis in Colombia have established collaborations with institutions in the Global North. This has allowed them to secure funding from both national and international agencies as well as attract individuals interested in health research in general.[2] Thus, recognizing that the amount of money allocated to science research in Colombia is still insufficient and among the lowest in Latin America (Ordóñez Matamoros et al. 2018; RICYT 2020, 25), some may argue that leishmaniasis has not been completely overlooked in terms of biomedical research. In what respect, then, can we talk about neglect in the case of Colombian leishmaniasis?

In this chapter, I discuss how neglect is particularly notorious in the omission of the armed conflict in the stories scientists tell about the disease in Colombia. These narratives insist on narrowly defining leishmaniasis as a biomedical problem with a pharmaceutical solution. I show that, although biomedical research and the armed conflict cannot be kept separate when studying a disease that primarily affects war zones, this connection is largely ignored in academic scientific articles. In fact, these papers discuss problems, observations, practices, results, and interpretations that are devoid of the violent context in which they are produced. Even though the war influences the everyday practices of leishmaniasis research, the narratives scientists create about the disease and their work on it have been, for the most part, "sanitized." In other words, the armed conflict, with all its dynamics, actors, and violence, has been filtered out to produce pacified accounts of science.

I argue this is partly a consequence of the neglected tropical diseases (NTDs) discourse, which frames diseases like leishmaniasis primarily as a problem of insufficient pharmaceuticals. This encourages scientists to narrow their focus to investigating pharmaceutical solutions. As a result, the vast majority of scientific research currently underway in Colombia seeks to identify better diagnostic tools and safer therapeutic options, as well as to understand why the available drugs often fail, how the biological action mechanisms behind these pharmaceuticals work, how patient compliance with these toxic medicines can be improved, and how to better follow up with patients during and after the treatment. By highlighting the lack of effective medications to treat leishmaniasis, most studies on the disease have fallen into the NTDs discursive trap. As a consequence, biomedical research narratives have rendered the war invisible, contributing to its neglect as the primary cause of leishmaniasis in Colombia. Thus, the pharmaceuticalization of both public health *and* biomedical research has obscured the central role played by the Colombian war in shaping the reality of leishmaniasis and contributed to further delaying the need to *desenmarañar* this disease from the war.

This final chapter is an attempt to partially redress that omission of war in the scientific narratives on leishmaniasis. I discuss war's place not only in our comprehension of the disease but also in the way we understand how the production of scientific knowledge about leishmaniasis takes place in Colombia. I do this with two main purposes. First, I want to draw attention to the enormous challenges and risks faced by scientists whose work involves chasing sandflies, detecting microscopic parasites, and collecting patient samples in war-torn areas among armed actors and civilians often surrounded by violence and illegal activities. Second, I want to begin a conversation about the implications of war's absence in the dominant narratives on leishmaniasis, especially regarding the "not-war-not-peace" situation (Nordstrom 2004) that characterizes Colombia's current political reality.

This chapter is organized into four sections. I start by discussing literature that examines the history of the NTD discourse and the global health strategies that emerge from it. Second, I highlight the persistence of the armed conflict in biomedical research on leishmaniasis by sharing the stories of Colombian scientists who have faced numerous hardships and risked their lives due to the circumstances surrounding their work. Third, I draw on ethnographic data collected at the Leishmaniasis Research Institute (LERI) clinic in Candelario to illustrate how leishmaniasis lesions and scars inevitably bring the war into the realm of biomedical knowledge production, revealing how science gets caught up in the *maraña*. Finally, I discuss how the NTDs discourse and scientists' claims of neutrality impact the role of scientific knowledge production in keeping war and leishmaniasis closely *enmarañados* in Colombia.

The Pharmaceuticalization of the Problem and Solution of NTDs

Jeremy Greene (2011) notes that by the mid-twentieth century, the role of prescription drugs in public health frameworks produced by international health organizations was much less salient than it is today. He explores "how the field of public health—which so frequently defined itself in opposition to biomedical approaches to disease—has now come to feature pharmaceutical delivery so prominently" (Greene 2011, 11). Highly attuned to the notion of the *pharmaceuticalization of public health* (Biehl 2007), Greene studied the genealogy of the "essential medicines" category and showed that pharmaceuticals went from being a negligible concern of public health practice to dominating the contemporary global health agenda since the 1970s. While acknowledging the importance of categorizing medicines as essential products, he cautions that "placing essential medicines at the center of global health priorities is not without its risks" (Greene 2011, 29). On the one hand, it reduces public health advocacy to pharmaceutical development and delivery. On the other, it repeats the same common mistake of understanding health in an overly narrow way as "the product of technical interventions divorced from economic, social, and political contexts" (Birn 2005, 515; see also McGoey 2015).

The discourse on NTDs follows the same pattern. It frames the problem of tropical diseases as a shortage of pharmaceutical interventions, which prevents non-drug-oriented solutions from being considered. Currently, leishmaniasis is one of twenty-two communicable diseases WHO defines as NTDs (WHO, n.d.), a label that emerged as a new disease category in the early 2000s (Vanderslott 2019). These include viral, helminthic, bacterial, and protozoal infections that are endemic in several tropical and subtropical countries mainly in Africa, Asia, and Latin America. Despite the broad diversity of these diseases, the narrative of neglect groups them together on the grounds that they disproportionately affect poor populations "who are less likely to have research directed for their benefit and where known interventions are limited by resources and not scaled up sufficiently" (Vanderslott 2019, 98). Therefore, establishing systems to develop and distribute medications for treating and preventing NTDs in impoverished regions is seen as the best approach. Following the example of the mass immunization campaigns of the 1980s, the response to NTDs has been drug-centered and "presented as morally appropriate, technically effective, and context-free" (M. Parker and Allen 2014, 223).

João Nunes writes that problem framing "is not merely a value-neutral exercise of identifying self-evident problems. Problems emerge as significant not just because they are 'there,' but also because they reinforce assumptions about what is important" (2016, 545). Thus, framing some diseases as neglected health issues shapes our perception in a way that reinforces beliefs about the relative importance of some problematic aspects while disregarding certain areas from the scope of concern (Nunes 2016). *Neglect* primarily refers to Big Pharma's historical lack of interest in developing medicines and vaccines for diseases affecting populations that do not represent a profitable market. This framing of neglect, in turn, has led to the idea that expanding access to pharmaceuticals as well as developing new drugs should dominate global health efforts to solve the lack of private companies' interest in these diseases (Greene 2011; Vanderslott 2019). As with other infectious diseases where drug delivery has turned into *the* public health strategy to control them (Biehl 2007), the pharmaceutical focus of NTD management is aligned with the more technological, disease-specific, and top-down approaches that, despite long-standing criticisms, continue to dominate global health (M. Parker and Allen 2014).

This framing has also pervaded the work of scientists doing research on NTDs. It has even come to significantly shape the practice of biomedical research in contexts where drug development capacities are limited and not necessarily the objective of scientific efforts. Such is the case of Colombian scientists conducting studies on leishmaniasis. They are currently directing most of their efforts toward antileishmanial drugs, turning their research into a pharmaceuticalized endeavor. Strategies based on molecular biology are considered paramount and dominate leishmaniasis research in Colombia. Consequently, the disease has become narrowly defined as a biomedical challenge, and the lack of effective drugs has taken over the definition of the problem posed by leishmaniasis.

The war remains unseen under this logic. As leishmaniasis scientists focus on what global health discourses on NTDs frame as problematic, drugs become dominant and deserving of concern, while the war disappears from their analysis of the disease. I asked my colleague Juan Pablo Centeno, a researcher at the Universidad Externado de Colombia, to help me illustrate this through a bibliometric analysis. He searched for articles on *Web of Science* that included the words *leishmaniasis* (or *leishmaniosis*) and *Colombia* in their titles, abstracts, and keywords. Of 21,489 results, only 1.57 percent included the terms *conflict*, *war*, *violence*, *guerrilla*, *military*, *army*, *soldier*, or *public order* between the years 2004 and 2022. This figure starkly illustrates the minimal role that the armed conflict plays in these scientific narratives.

War cannot be easily accommodated within the narrative of NTDs. While much of the focus revolves around the market's indifference toward the health problems of impoverished people, this discourse tends to overlook how violence and conflict disproportionately affect and sicken them. In other words, problematizing an illness as a neglected tropical disease does little to explain how war can shape, in distinctive and critical ways, the epidemiological patterns, therapeutic itineraries, and lived experiences of a particular disease. Without fully considering the *maraña* formed by leishmaniasis and the armed conflict, biomedical research has inadvertently neglected the major social determinant of the disease in the Colombian context. The NTDs discourse has become a trap that has led to the pharmaceuticalization of both public health and biomedical research, all while obscuring the central role the war has played in shaping the reality of Colombian leishmaniasis.

Drawing on Michael Taussig's (1999) notion of *public secrets*, Paul Wenzel Geissler (2013) shows that actively "unknowing" known facts about the reality in which health research unfolds helps produce scientific knowledge amid, and despite, multiple inequalities and contradictions. He asks "how (and why) a group of people that is brought together by the scientific pursuit of truth with a view of transforming both knowledge and, through it, the world, retains—indeed creates—zones of unknowing at the core of its practices" (Geissler 2013, 16). Geissler is more concerned with the differences in material living conditions between study participants and research staff, and how these are handled in day-to-day research work but are left out of scientific texts and public speech. I, however, find his analysis highly valuable in illuminating the omission of the armed conflict from the official narratives of leishmaniasis created by Colombian scientists. Inspired by his work, I explore why scientists come to "unknow" certain aspects of leishmaniasis while researching and writing about the scientific facts of this disease.

Navigating the Dangers of Leishmaniasis Research

As I mentioned in chapter 1, the largest leishmaniasis outbreak documented in Colombia was in Chaparral, Tolima, between 2003 and 2006. Entomologists, biologists, biomedical scientists, clinicians, epidemiologists, and public health specialists from Bogotá, Medellín, and Cali saw in the Chaparral epidemic an important opportunity for further leishmaniasis research.[3] Among this group was Martín Mejía, a biologist with almost thirty years of experience in investigating how sandflies and mammals exchange *Leishmania* parasites. Martín's master's thesis was part of a much larger scientific project exploring clinical and environmental aspects of the leishmaniasis outbreak in Chaparral. Due to his interest in animals, especially the numerous species involved in what scientists call "the leishmaniasis transmission cycle," Martín spent most of his time doing fieldwork at the homes of peasants living in rural areas of the municipality. However, guerrilla members of the Fuerzas Armadas Revolucionarias de Colombia (FARC) eventually approached him and told him that he was not allowed in those areas. Martín described his experience to me: "They [the FARC] would tell you only once. I could not take the risk, so the [research] process stopped for six months—there was a delay in the project timeline. Then, I started figuring out a solution. It was an individual solution, not an institutional solution. You were trying to save your own *pellejo* [save your neck], save my thesis, the project. I had to solve the situation. So, at that moment, I said 'I have to talk to people in the community who are in contact with [guerrillas] and know them . . . and get a mediator.' "

The "mediator" ended up being a man from one of the peasant families with whom Martín had developed a close relationship. That past December, Martín had wanted to do something festive for the community, so he gathered the children from this man's family and others to put up a Christmas tree and build a traditional nativity scene. At that time, however, he could not have imagined that this kind gesture would play a vital role in the continuation of his research project. The man agreed to help Martín and scheduled an appointment with the FARC commander who was operating in that area. Martín and his friend drove four hours up the mountain for the meeting, which Martín described to me as follows:

> For me, it was humiliating that I, a Colombian, had to ask another Colombian to let me work in my country. I felt uncomfortable, but, at the same time, I had to accept the situation. [Right before the meeting] I had to wait for a while in a line because other people also had appointments with the commander. Then, I was told to come in. The guy [the guerrilla commander] was sitting behind a table . . . I tried to explain to him that we were identifying [leishmaniasis] risk factors, and we wanted to see how the transmission was taking place there. He responded with a series of ill-founded, false theories. He said that there had never been leishmaniasis in that area before,[4] that it was actually the Army who had released the disease there, and that that was how people had started to get sick.[5] "That's valid," I said to him. "But let me prove another theory from the academic standpoint, from what we know. I know you know that there are insects that bite and transmit diseases. Let me look into that." Probably because I was with the other guy [the mediator], the commander finally accepted. . . . He told me "You have to give me your name, your identification number, and the list of the houses you are visiting and the people who live in them. And if we ever need you, you have to be available." I told him that was not a problem . . . I carried on working because I had to finish gathering my data. That could not be interrupted indefinitely, the project couldn't stop either.

Like many other researchers who study leishmaniasis in Colombia, Martín was forced to confront the rules, power dynamics, and logic of war head-on. When I asked leishmaniasis scientists about the dangers they had experienced during their research, they usually shared stories about dangerous situations and fear-inspiring events involving guerrilla and paramilitary groups, as well as members of the Army. In Colombia, leishmaniasis research does not merely involve the expected challenges faced by those who study the vector-borne diseases that affect people in marginal, dispersed, and remote areas. In this context, conducting research on leishmaniasis can be risky and require negotiating work conditions with armed actors who are often seen as authorities in areas where the disease and the war are endemic (see Arjona 2016).

Leishmaniasis researchers say that, regardless of the conflict, the right to health must prevail. Beyond their political convictions, they see themselves as neutral actors who claim not to take sides in the social and armed conflict that has shaped Colombia for more than six decades. The words of Armando Ospina are illustrative of this point. He is a physician and epidemiologist with ten years of experience developing leishmaniasis research projects, most of them carried out in southwestern Colombia. I asked if he had ever encountered members of armed groups, and this was his response: "I know that they [armed actors] are there, I know that I have provided medical care for them, but I don't ask those questions. I know it's them—I mean, I have a sense of it. And I don't ask any more questions so I don't have more information about anything. I am treating the human being; adjectives do not enter into my analysis. But I have had to deal with everyone, with all of them, with everyone."

Humanitarian notions of health and biomedical research permeate these claims of neutrality. They operate as guarantors of impartiality and objectivity and as protective measures against acts of direct violence that might endanger researchers. Armando prefers not to know the story behind the leishmaniasis ulcers of his patients so as to protect science—and himself—from the corrosive effects of war. In this case, claims to objectivity and neutrality are a useful political tool to navigate the perils and complexities of the *enmarañamiento* between field research and war. However, it remains undeniable that war provides the overarching backdrop for this scientific work.

When War Is the Context of Biomedical Research

Candelario's downtown is home to a small clinic that belongs to LERI, whose administrative offices and laboratories are located hundreds of kilometers away in one of Colombia's largest cities. In the world of biomedical research, LERI has earned national and international renown and credibility based on the prolific publication of studies on leishmaniasis that have received support from funding agencies promoting health research in Colombia and abroad. This clinic has been in Candelario since the early 1980s, and most of LERI's leishmaniasis research relies on patients and communities affected by the disease in rural areas of this municipality.

Initially, LERI's work was more interventionist and oriented toward public health. Research staff actively searched for leishmaniasis cases in Candelario's rural areas. They carried microscopes, medical supplies, and Glucantime ampoules to diagnose and treat the disease and also collected biological samples, counted cases, and mapped patient distribution. In the mid-1990s, with the collaboration of departmental and municipal health authorities, LERI expanded these interventions to extremely remote areas that could only be reached by boat through several rivers. However, in the late 1990s and early 2000s, the armed conflict reached Candelario, and LERI had to reduce its field interventions.

As a central component of the US-Colombia antidrug policy, the use of military aircraft to fumigate and eradicate coca plantations became widespread in the south of the country, primarily in the *departamentos* of Putumayo, Caquetá, and Meta (Ramírez 2011; Ciro Rodríguez 2020). Under these conditions, a significant portion of the cocaine production and business did not decrease but instead moved to the Pacific region, reaching places like Candelario, where the conflict had only had a minimal presence up to that point. The drug production involved the influx of armed actors and drug trafficking networks, the militarization of Candelario, and the arrival of large numbers of peasant families whose survival depended on the harvesting and processing of coca leaves. The racial landscape also changed. A population largely made up of the descendants of Africans brought to the Americas in the transatlantic slave trade now came to be composed of mestizos (people of mixed European and Indigenous ancestry) from other regions of Colombia. Since then, Candelario has turned into a battleground and a hub for cocaine production, and violence is a persistent element of everyday life, primarily in rural zones.

In response, LERI's work became increasingly limited to biomedical research projects that relied on molecular biology technologies that could be conducted within the safety of laboratory walls. These changes in LERI's work occurred at the same time as the emergence of the global health discourse on NTDs and shifts in biomedical research that led to the "molecular takeover of medicine." Along with the rise of gene technology, these developments produced increasingly molecularized and lab-based understandings of diseases and their possible cures (Rheinberger 2000, 20). The few research initiatives that continued to be developed in rural areas had to adapt to ensure both the safety of LERI's staff and the feasibility of the projects. In other words, the armed conflict changed the way researchers could enter the field. Some of the strategies included notifying the health authorities and, in many cases, the local authorities (military and/or nonstate armed groups) in advance; seeking the participation of local residents in the research teams, ideally someone from the local health service; and carrying a Medical Mission card and vest to identify research and health personnel as a way of enforcing compliance with international humanitarian law.

From that point on, the responsibilities of LERI staff in Candelario gradually shifted toward only evaluating people who came to the clinic with skin lesions. Their eligibility was determined by whether they met the inclusion criteria of the now predominantly molecular biology–based projects that LERI researchers were working on. Those who did were diagnosed with and treated for leishmaniasis in accordance with the national CPG (fig. 5.1). In

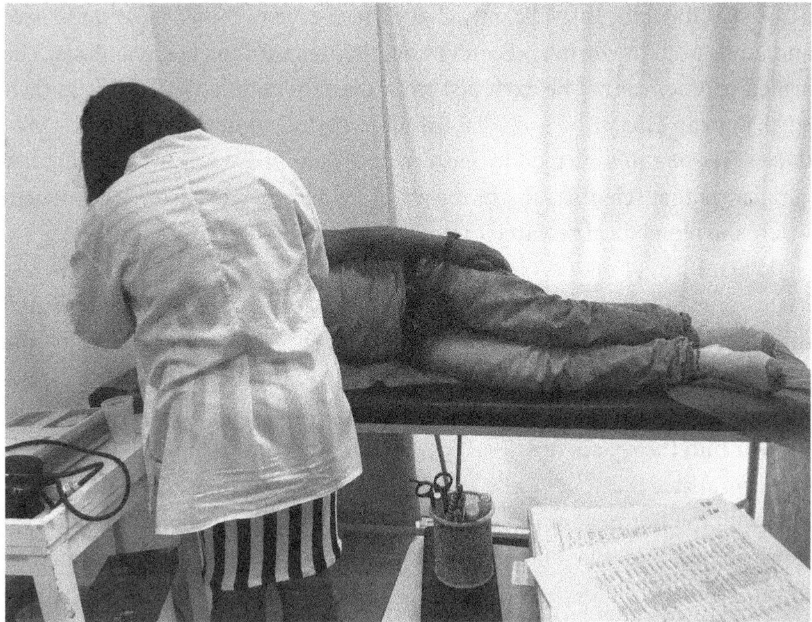

FIGURE 5.1. Doctor examining a leishmaniasis patient at the LERI clinic in Candelario. Photo by Lina Pinto-García.

return, leishmaniasis patients were asked to become research subjects. If they accepted, consent forms were signed, and data and biological samples were collected and sent digitally and by air to LERI's main facility. There, the information and materials served as indispensable resources for the development of various projects, many of which were focused on basic biomedical research, while others guided public health decisions.

Both war and changes in global health discourses and biomedical research practices have significantly shaped the type of work done by scientific institutions interested in leishmaniasis in Colombia. The example of LERI shows that the armed conflict has impacted not only the logistics of conducting research projects but also the type of research questions posed by scientists. However, as I mention below, these changes are also due to and intertwined with the progressive pharmaceuticalization of global health, which makes drugs central to the biomedical research of NTDs.

In the following section, I show that, in the everyday work of leishmaniasis research in Colombia, war is an unavoidable, persistent, and central element of scientific practice. In other words, I describe how the armed conflict and its associated dynamics significantly shape the everyday context that influences and limits both the form and content of scientific work on leishmaniasis. The armed conflict cannot be excluded from the production of scientific knowledge, nor can science be excluded from the violent context in which it is produced. The *maraña* formed by leishmaniasis and the war is not confined to rural areas that scientists might regard as field sites. It exists in other spaces where the biomedical research on this disease takes place.

When I was at the Candelario clinical facility, I was able to trace how the leishmaniasis lesions and biological samples that constitute the fundamental raw material of biomedical research are, for the most part, produced by the everyday war dynamics that prevail in rural areas and conflict zones. Drawing on this ethnographic data, I contend that leishmaniasis inevitably pulls the war into the spaces of scientific research. Those who move leishmaniasis from rural areas into scientific spaces are the people whose lives are entangled with the war in complex and varied ways. As scientific practice relies on those people, scientific knowledge on leishmaniasis is also deeply immersed in the *maraña*.

DISPLACEMENT, COCA HARVESTING, AND LEISHMANIASIS ULCERS

In March of 2017, Tulia and her seventeen-year-old son Alejandro arrived at the LERI clinic in Candelario. Unlike most of the residents of this municipality, the woman and her son were not Afro-Colombians. At the reception desk, Alejandro showed two ulcers on his right elbow to Juliana, one of the nursing assistants. One was larger than the other, and both were circular, with raised edges and a scab in the center—they looked like textbook leishmaniasis lesions. Juliana led him to a small room. Pointing at a stretcher, she asked him to lie on his left side so she could collect the samples that would allow her to diagnose the disease. Juliana put on latex gloves and cleaned the lesions with an iodized solution. She used her left hand to pinch the skin of the patient's elbow. Holding a scalpel in her right hand, she "scraped" the edges of the lesions sideways.[6] When Juliana was satisfied with the fluid she had collected, she spread the sample over a microscope slide, drawing a bloody and watery circle with the scalpel blade. She repeated this process several times until she had two slides, each with three samples. She gave the young man a clean gauze and told him to press it firmly against the lesions to stop the bleeding and ease the pain caused by the procedure. After taking the slides to another room, she used a purple solution (Giemsa stain) to dye the samples, then allowed them to dry before looking at them through the microscope for

Leishmania parasites. In the meantime, Alejandro and his mother met with Diana, one of LERI's physicians.

Alejandro and Tulia told us they lived in a rural area an hour's drive from the urban center of Candelario. Despite being treated with herbal plasters for four months, Alejandro's lesions had not healed and continued to grow. Therefore, they decided to go to LERI on the recommendation of several people. In an effort to find out where he had contracted leishmaniasis, I asked Alejandro if he spent a lot of time in forested areas. He nodded timidly while looking at the floor, and Tulia told us that he worked *en la raspa* (harvesting coca leaves), in *fincas* (farms) deep inside the jungle, about two hours away from where they lived. He wasn't the only one. The whole family had the same job, including Tulia and her six other children. Overcoming his shyness, Alejandro told us he was used to staying at those farms for up to fifteen days at a time. I asked him if he was going to school. "He went to school up to seventh grade but didn't want to go anymore," Tulia replied. She went on to say that in the places where they worked, she had seen several people with *guaral*, as leishmaniasis is locally known. "There's a lot of that mosquito over there. Most people get cured using plants. It works for some, but not for others," she said (see Pinto-García 2025).

Suspecting that they were not originally from Candelario, I asked Tulia where they had come from. Alejandro had been born and raised in Candelario, but she had grown up in a town in Putumayo. Tulia was one of the many peasants who had migrated to the Colombian Pacific region because of the extensive use of herbicides to eradicate coca plants in that *departamento*. That is how she and the rest of her family ended up in Candelario in the early 2000s. Their lives continued to be affected by war in devastating ways. She told us that guerrillas had killed two brothers and seven nieces and nephews. As if this were not enough, she was left homeless when her house was seized by the military during armed confrontations between the Army and the FARC, and the guerrillas responded by throwing two improvised mortars against the building. Neither side took responsibility.

As Diana and I listened attentively to this heartbreaking succession of tragedies, Juliana came into the office and confirmed that she had detected *Leishmania* parasites in the samples taken from Alejandro's ulcers. Diana asked Alejandro and Tulia if they would agree to his participation in a follow-up research study that LERI was conducting at that time. If they accepted, a person without formal training but with experience as local health promoter would visit them once a week to evaluate the healing process of Alejandro's leishmaniasis lesions and monitor his symptoms during and after Glucantime treatment. That information would then be recorded through a mobile app developed by LERI researchers to monitor the treatment and recovery of patients with leishmaniasis. They agreed, and Diana asked Tulia to sign several consent forms to formalize Alejandro's enrollment in the study. Tulia was given a plastic bag with six boxes, each one containing ten ampoules of Glucantime, and a record sheet to write down the amount of medication administered to Alejandro daily. On the back of the sheet, Diana wrote *Sulfaplata*, a cream Alejandro needed to use on the lesions to avoid secondary bacterial infection. She also explained how Glucantime was to be administered daily: split the contents of three ampoules into two injections, 6 ml for one buttock and 7 ml for the other. Leftovers were to be discarded. Diana asked Tulia and Alejandro to keep the empty vials of Glucantime and give them to the person who was going to follow up on the treatment. Tulia and Alejandro thanked Diana, said goodbye, and left the clinic.

Tulia and Alejandro's story is hardly exceptional. It is actually very similar to many of the accounts I heard at LERI's clinic. As Alejandro entered this scientific space with his leishmaniasis lesions, he brought with him the complex realities of the armed conflict, the violence, and the inequitable conditions of rural Colombia these ulcers carried with them. Since leishmaniasis and war are deeply *enmarañados*, the disease inevitably brings the war into the research facility. When leishmaniasis occupies the spaces of scientific research, war comes along with it and becomes impossible to ignore. Yet scientists overlook the conflict in their published work on leishmaniasis.

WAR ULCERS

In February of 2017, two men visited the LERI clinic in Candelario. One was around sixty, short with black skin. He was wearing a blue cap, shorts, and a red T-shirt, and he had a thick Candelarian accent. The other man was mestizo, tall and younger. He wore a yellow T-shirt with English inscriptions, jeans, a thin poncho over his shoulder, and a small leather bag. His cap had an equestrian motif, and his red sneakers looked brand-new. The older man said he had already had leishmaniasis and showed Juliana a testimonial scar on his right arm. Because he was familiar with LERI from his previous experience, he said, he had brought his friend in to have an ulcer checked.

The younger man's name was Gerardo. He was from a town in Meta and had arrived in Candelario several months earlier. I asked him why he came. "To visit," he replied curtly. Another man joined Gerardo and the older man. He called Gerardo "boss," and Gerardo gave him orders to buy some items while he was at LERI. The man left once he understood all his tasks.

Gerardo had a large, elongated ulcer on the lower part of his belly. He also had a small scar on his arm from another lesion that had healed. He told me that he was familiar with leishmaniasis but had never contracted the disease until he came to Candelario. Aurora, one of the nursing assistants, asked if he had put anything on the ulcer. "Yes, of course," he replied. Initially, he said, he had used topical antibiotics. Later, he admitted to having applied a mixture of urine, tobacco, and some kind of crushed pill. At one point, he had been injected with penicillin. Sitting in front of a computer, Aurora asked for his full name and identification number to enter this information into a database. When she asked for his cell phone number, Gerardo became somewhat anxious and said it would be better to write down his friend's number because his own cell phone had permanent connection problems. Aurora insisted that LERI needed a number where he could be reached. Gerardo finally gave her a number and said it was his sister's, who was in Bogotá but with whom he communicated regularly. Several minutes later, Aurora once more demanded that Gerardo give her the number of the cell phone he was holding. He finally agreed. While waiting for one of LERI's doctors to see him, Gerardo told Aurora and me that leishmaniasis was "the second enemy of the state." "First the guerrillas and then leishmaniasis," he said. He told us he had read that in a newspaper. Indeed, newspaper articles have often portrayed leishmaniasis as yet another enemy of the Colombian Army (for instance, *El Tiempo* 2005b, 2007, 2005a).

During the medical consultation, a physician named Mauricio told Gerardo that LERI was running a study that compared different sampling methods to diagnose leishmaniasis. He invited Gerardo to participate, and he agreed without much fuss. Mauricio had Gerardo complete and sign an informed consent form, asked some questions, and entered data into the computer. A software program developed by LERI randomized the order in which four different sampling procedures were to be carried out. Aurora and another nursing assistant, Jairo, directed Gerardo to a small room and had him lie down on the stretcher and remove his T-shirt. They started with the smear. Jairo unpacked a blade and scraped the edges of the ulcer, causing it to bleed. Gerardo made sudden, involuntary movements and complained of pain. Jairo spread the sample on a pair of microscope slides that he passed to Aurora. He then unpacked two swabs and rubbed them against the inner edges of the lesion. Gerardo jumped in agony, complaining about the pain and taking a deep breath through his teeth. After dipping the bloodstained swabs into a buffer solution, Jairo inserted a tiny screw into the edge of the ulcer, turned it, and removed it. Gerardo protested, but not as much as he had with the swabs. The sample was also suspended in a buffer solution. Finally, Jairo took two small syringes containing a few milliliters of antibiotic solution. He punctured the edge of the lesion and moved the plunger up and over with twisting motions several times. He repeated the procedure with the other syringe. Aurora took the syringes to another room, lit a burner to avoid microbial contamination, and deposited the samples in four test tubes containing red culture medium. On a sheet of paper depicting a pain scale with a line, Gerardo classified the four procedures from the least to the most painful.

The sample taken with the screw came back positive. The swab test was invalid. Aurora phoned the principal investigators at LERI to ask if she should repeat the procedure and was told not to. As for the samples taken with syringes, the cultures were kept in an incubator and sent to LERI's main laboratory a few days later. The smear also came back positive: *Leishmania* parasites could be seen under the microscope. Mauricio confirmed to Gerardo that he indeed had leishmaniasis and gave him all the Glucantime ampoules he needed in a yellow bag.

When Gerardo and his companion left the clinic, I asked Mauricio what he thought about him. "He must be part of one of those [armed] groups," he replied. Then he showed me one of the forms Mauricio had filled out. In the space for the patient's occupation, he had written *agricultor* (farmer). "I can't put *paraco* [paramilitary]," he said, implying what he (and I) actually suspected about Gerardo. If the patient was involved in trafficking cocaine, Mauricio said, writing *agricultor* was not entirely false.

People with vague affiliations often visit LERI's clinic to seek medical care for their skin lesions. They may be guerrillas, paramilitaries, armed actors who are not clearly one or the other, drug traffickers, or workers involved in cocaine production or illegal mining. Some might simply be civilians living in areas where conflict and its impacts are daily occurrences. Yet when they come to LERI, all of them become patients and potential research subjects. Whether they are civilians, members of armed groups, or people involved in illegal activities, research staff believe that the right to health prevails.

However, unintended consequences arise. Even though leishmaniasis lesions develop amid and because of the war and its associated economies, the biological samples and data collected by LERI employees are transformed into context-free materials and information for biomedical research. Although leishmaniasis is deeply *enmarañado* with the armed conflict and pulls this violent reality into scientific spaces, the practices used to generate knowledge under NTDs discourses of global health separate the war and the disease, the latter of which becomes depoliticized and decontextualized. This misleading separation is evident in scientists' accounts, in which leishmaniasis is characterized as a health issue affecting communities on the margins of the economy—a problem that could be solved with more effective pharmaceutical products capable of "end[ing] diseases of poverty, and maybe poverty itself" (M. Parker and Allen 2014, 224).

Pharmaceuticalized Research and the Omission of War

Most of the research on leishmaniasis in Colombia has fallen into the NTDs discursive trap, which portrays the lack of effective pharmaceuticals as the most critical aspect of solving this health problem. In light of this reasoning, scientists have shifted their focus from public health frameworks and toward research questions related to diagnostic and therapeutic tools as well as molecular aspects relevant to the efficacy of these technologies. Yolanda Paredes, a microbiologist who has researched leishmaniasis at a public university for thirty years, explained the situation:

> Many of the researchers who are getting trained are being trained through scientific papers, right? Obviously, what's taught in graduate school is that you have to be up to date—you have to be up to date with the latest information, right? . . . And since I'm working on leishmaniasis, I started doing the same thing [as the research article says]. This [approach] results in researchers who have never had contact with a leishmaniasis patient. Many of these researchers don't have basic epidemiological knowledge. And I'm not talking about the epidemiological knowledge that involves repeating global leishmaniasis statistics, no. I am referring to the knowledge of the reality of the disease in rural areas of the country.

Some scientists who specialize in leishmaniasis are so immersed in their laboratory research that they have little to no interaction with patients. In order to secure funding and stay relevant, they do not need to know the context from which samples and data come. They also do not need to be aware of the impact of war on patients' lives or the conditions under which they became infected with *Leishmania*. Despite the significant influence of armed conflict on the production of scientific knowledge, pacified depictions of science remain the norm in academic literature. Although war is a common aspect of most leishmaniasis studies, especially in patient recruitment and the collection of biological materials for biomedical research, scientists rarely mention the conflict in their writings. This disregard persists even when the violence of war constrains how scientific knowledge on leishmaniasis is produced.

Scientists have faced many difficulties, risked their careers, and put themselves in danger for doing their job. This is especially true for those whose work is not confined to the labs. The war has delayed, changed, or canceled their research projects. Due to the changing cartography and unfolding history of the armed conflict, scientists often navigate shifting conditions that compel them to select work areas perceived as safer or to adopt security measures they deem appropriate and sufficient for the circumstances at hand. They sometimes must negotiate their movements within rural areas with armed actors—Army, guerrillas, and paramilitaries. Remarkably, however, many scientists continue their leishmaniasis research despite the associated risks. Persuaded that it is worthwhile to continue working despite the war, many scientists believe that producing knowledge and evidence on leishmaniasis is necessary to transform the unequal distribution of the burden of disease and reduce health disparities. Researchers have regularly sought the company of local public health workers and community members who live in endemic areas because these people sometimes manage to legitimize the presence of the outsiders. Often, locals are able to provide scientists with a certain level of protection while they collect sandflies, take biological samples, distribute mosquito nets, give talks on leishmaniasis, recruit patients for clinical studies, or administer antileishmanial medicines. Nevertheless, the risks have never fully disappeared.

Scientists tend to ignore the violent environment in which their work takes place when it comes to publishing research. War and violence are treated as "externalities" in scientific work. They are irrelevant when making the sort of generalizations about pharmaceutical technologies that the NTD discursive game expects to hear. This disregard of the armed conflict is even more striking in scientific publications in which the subjects' backgrounds cannot be disassociated from the war. Such is the case of the individuals visiting the LERI clinic in Candelario and the soldiers receiving treatment for leishmaniasis at the CRL. In many other contexts and historical periods, military personnel have participated in medical research (Newlands 2013; Baader et al. 2005). Scientific studies on leishmaniasis conducted in Colombia have relied on this population, which includes hundreds of Army soldiers chosen as research subjects for biomedical research projects, clinical studies, and clinical trials on leishmaniasis (for instance, López et al. 2013, 2018; Patino et al. 2017; Perez-Franco et al. 2016). Soldiers do not only provide the bodies to fight the state war against guerrilla organizations; they also volunteer their bodies to scientific research on leishmaniasis.

The involvement of military and nonmilitary patients in these studies, whose lives are marked in various ways by the armed conflict, demonstrates the intricate *maraña* that holds war and leishmaniasis research together. It also serves as a poignant example of how science and war mutually shape each other in a context of violence. Undeniably, participation in these studies has allowed some patients to receive treatments that are less harmful than Glucantime and that would otherwise have been inaccessible to them. Nevertheless, it is important to emphasize that the development of scientific knowledge on leishmaniasis in Colombia has heavily relied on the armed conflict. This includes the participation of soldiers in clinical studies, as well as the violent conditions under which civilian study participants contract the disease in rural areas. Despite these realities, scientific articles do not explore or acknowledge this close relationship between war and the study subjects. In the case of soldiers, military affiliation is often mentioned only in passing within the articles' methods section, where study subjects are typically described very briefly. However, the broader implications of warfare for scientific practices and results are not discussed, and the mutual influence and reinforcement of technoscience and the armed conflict remains unquestioned.

The pacified accounts of science published by leishmaniasis researchers reveal the deeply political character of neutrality claims. Neutrality may be a way to navigate the contradictions of war in order to carry out research. At the same time, disavowing the violent roots of the disease and downplaying their relevance under pharmaceuticalized accounts of the problem only serves to maintain and reinforce the *maraña* formed by war and leishmaniasis.

Acting as the spokespersons and representatives of leishmaniasis and leishmaniasis patients, scientists have inadvertently contributed to the invisibility of the war in the collective understanding of both the disease and the way research on leishmaniasis is produced. By insisting that tropical diseases are biomedical problems that could be solved if effective and safe drugs were available, the war (and peace building) is rarely mentioned in the analysis of the issue and the strategies used to address it. Constrained by global health agendas and the perspective of the NTDs discourse on leishmaniasis, scientists find it unnecessary, potentially risky or outside the scope of their discipline to account for the war that affects and pervades their work. As a result, their daily struggles are misrepresented through narratives that obscure how scientists themselves navigate the dangers of researching leishmaniasis. Despite the *maraña* formed by war and leishmaniasis, and the impact of the armed conflict on scientific work, the pharmaceuticalization of leishmaniasis research in Colombia has created a distorted view of the problem, hindering efforts to disentangle the structural and historical factors of this complex relationship.

Conclusion

A partial tree trunk stands in what appeared to be the geographic center of the Colinas ZVNT—one of the twenty-six locations designated for the concentration and disarmament of FARC members after the signing of the peace agreement. A small white flag on a thin wooden pole is held in the trunk's cracks. Though somewhat dusty, the square piece of cloth is made of a silky and shiny material—perhaps from an elegant garment like a bridal gown or a first communion dress. As the hems were already worn down, the edges had begun to fray, and each gust of wind threatened to disintegrate the fabric. Someone had used a black marker to carefully write three capital letters in the center: P-A-Z. *PAZ*. PEACE (fig. 6.1).

Every time I think of this modest monument, I imagine a former guerrilla feeling the impulse—the need—to mark the point at which the signing of the peace deal became a significant part of Colombia's history. Throughout this period of transition, which commenced with the successful conclusion of the peace negotiations in Havana, I have often thought of this flag as a nearly perfect representation of the uncertain times and ambivalent emotions that most FARC ex-combatants and many other Colombians—like myself—had experienced. For me, that precarious yet imposing peace symbol has come to capture the ups and downs of the present situation. At present, peace in Colombia is a remarkable but highly fragile achievement. Peace is polished, clear, and coherent on paper, but convoluted, unfinished, and contradictory in reality. Peace requires high doses of both hope and skepticism in order to be made and remade on a daily basis. Peace did not make us a better or fairer country overnight. Nor has peace put us on a straightforward path to become a less violent or more democratic nation. However, the almost four years of peace negotiations between the FARC and the state, as well as the

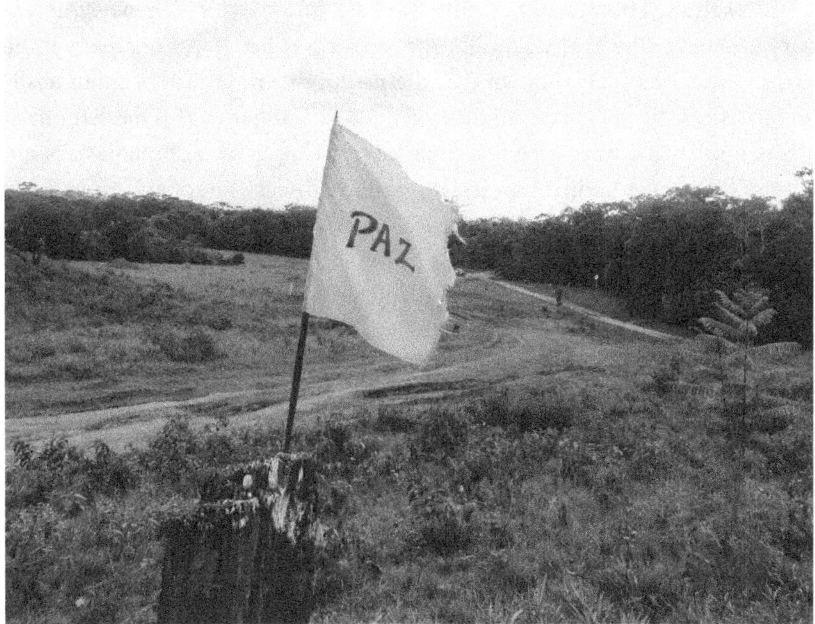

FIGURE 6.1. Flag raised in the middle of the Colinas disarmament camp in Guaviare. Photo by Lina Pinto-García.

more than seven years of the peace agreement implementation, have made us more aware of the challenges ahead. I think it is fair to say that we are now better positioned to acknowledge what peace implies, what the aspirations of a nonviolent country demand. We are now much more cautious in estimating how much remains to be done.

Part of that caution involves building a deep understanding of the ubiquitous and inescapable nature of war and recognizing that the armed conflict has penetrated every sociocultural corner of Colombian society. With the goal of tracing the complex connections between disease and violence, this book offers an ethnographic narrative aligned with what Didier Fassin calls a *politics of recognition*, which, "as opposed to a politics of denial, implies both identifying and naming violence, affirming its existence where it is ignored, and giving it a reality by speaking of it" (2009, 117). As such, this work has shown that when warfare and militarization are pervasive, violence spreads everywhere, engulfing even the actors, objects, discourses, and good intentions of biomedical research, medical practice, and public health.

Throughout this book, I have asserted that contending seriously with the problem of leishmaniasis in Colombia requires keeping the war at the center of the analysis. This means bringing war back into the story whenever necessary, whenever the armed conflict is portrayed as being just one part of the larger issue. I have also shown that the predominant narratives about leishmaniasis in Colombia have minimized the role of the war. This has left unaddressed the many ways in which the suffering caused by leishmaniasis is not always due to the bodily manifestation of the disease but often results from the entanglement between the physical marks left on the skin and the ideas and practices of biomedicine, public health, and the armed conflict.

In this work, I have shown that war and leishmaniasis have formed an intricate and messy *maraña* that entangles, through multiple processes and mechanisms, a broad range of actors, institutions, types of knowledge, forms of logic, practices, and technologies. Leishmaniasis is not simply a side effect of the war. Nor is violent conflict a separate entity affecting leishmaniasis's natural course from the outside. On the contrary, this disease and "all the [other] effects of war violence inhabit the same plane" (MacLeish 2013, 9). War and leishmaniasis are not two separate phenomena that circumstantially encounter each other when combatants enter the jungle, get bitten by sandflies, and leave these forested environments with growing skin ulcers. Instead, the experience of leishmaniasis in Colombia for all those affected by the disease—not only soldiers, guerrillas, or paramilitaries—is shaped by the armed conflict in many ways. In a similar vein, war is also enacted through leishmaniasis, especially when a person's access to medical care and antileishmanial drugs depends on his status in relation to the logic and social divisions caused by the war. Leishmaniasis in Colombia shows how society and technoscience influence each other in a violent context, creating and reproducing warfare systems of health and illness that divide people into allies and excluded enemies.

What this disease tells us about the conflict in Colombia is that war spreads everywhere; that violence invokes and engages unanticipated actors and mechanisms; and that to overcome the armed conflict and achieve peace, it is not enough to address only the obvious expressions and consequences of war. Instead, achieving peace requires delving into war's thick layers, which are deeply rooted in ordinary life and intertwined in human and more-than-human worlds. I have included phrases that are useful in ensuring that the impact of war is not ignored in how we understand leishmaniasis. They are also meant to support epidemiological discussions that, although they define the armed conflict as a social determinant of this disease, fail to explain the processes through which this relationship is produced and maintained. Finally, they aim to question global health views that easily and almost automatically blame all that is wrong with leishmaniasis—in Colombia and elsewhere—on its "neglected tropical disease" status.

First, speaking of *Colombian leishmaniasis* forces us to carefully consider the local particularities, historical trajectories, and geopolitics of knowledge that make leishmaniasis in Colombia so distinctive because of its *enmarañamiento* with the war. As Michael Westerhaus has noted, ignoring the crucial role that violence plays in the transmission and suffering linked to certain infectious diseases "risks the formation of an acontextual narrative with questionable accuracy" (2007, 595). Thus, I have emphasized that speaking of leishmaniasis as *a disease of war* is helpful to shift the focus to the *maraña* and stay close to its deeply enmeshed connections to the armed conflict until a different—and hopefully less violent—relationship can be established.

Secondly, I use *pharmaceuticalization of war* as a term to conceptualize the mechanisms and practices through which pharmaceuticals are made into strategic war-making technologies in response to rationales and social orders produced by the armed conflict. Health access barriers are not "natural occurrences." They do not emerge from one day to the other, widening the gap between the sick and the cure. Obstacles between individuals and the fulfillment of their rights are created along power structures whose disposition and rigidity depend on historical processes. The war in Colombia has played a key role in the current political architecture that puts some above others and justifies violence against certain populations. Among many other imbalances, the war has created a situation where both guerrillas and civilians in rural areas are left for the most part untreated for a disease that worsens these inequities. In contrast, soldiers of the Colombian Army represent the only group of people with full and guaranteed access to Glucantime, the pharmaceutical traditionally used to manage leishmaniasis in Colombia. Yet the imperative to ensure that as many soldiers as possible are ready to fight the war—at any cost—has positioned this drug at the center of a therapeutic system where military bodies slowly deteriorate and finally become disposable.

By combining these ideas, I hope to have convinced the reader that the *desenmarañamiento* of leishmaniasis and the armed conflict should not be framed as a biomedical problem with a pharmaceutical solution. As Beth Linker writes, it is an illusion to think "that the human ravages of war [can] be erased with a technological fix" (2011, 7). In other words, pharmaceuticalizing the solution is not the answer either. Eliminating the access barriers to Glucantime may seem like *the* way to solve the issue, but only simplifies the problem. It also overlooks the complex nature of the *maraña* and the war-related experience of Colombian leishmaniasis. Although crucial, ensuring access to antileishmanial therapies—ideally free of antimony and other toxic compounds—is only one of the many ways to start repairing the violence that leishmaniasis sufferers must experience. However, focusing only on this issue would mean ignoring the harm caused by Glucantime and other antileishmanial pharmaceuticals, damage that has been borne out by the bodies of Colombian soldiers. Even if new biomedical technologies were developed to prevent or treat leishmaniasis, their use in Colombia would most likely follow the same lines of Glucantime distribution, leading to the same violent patterns of inclusion and exclusion, and leaving the stigmatization of leishmaniasis sufferers as guerrilla members unchallenged.

I have tried to engage with complexity by paying careful attention to some of the multiple threads that hold the *maraña* together. In an attempt to link theory, analysis, and critique to practice, I want to briefly reflect on how some of the problematic elements that I have revealed lead to possibilities of intervention to reduce the harm caused by leishmaniasis in Colombia. What can we do to start *desenmarañando* war and leishmaniasis? How can this book motivate the community, medical facilities, and the government to implement policies that will reduce the suffering of people affected by this disease? First, I believe it is important to develop strategies to destigmatize the disease at different levels. In places where the stigma of "the guerrilla disease" persists, it is crucial to take specific actions to identify and challenge the mindset of "friend or enemy" whenever it endangers the well-being and safety of those with leishmaniasis ulcers. To this end, it is important to work at the community level, in clinical facilities, and within public health and military institutions.

Second, it is imperative to change how Glucantime is administered to all patients with leishmaniasis in Colombia. As I have argued elsewhere (Pinto-García 2022), this drug should be used only when there are no other suitable treatment options. During the conflict, FARC guerrilla members who had medical responsibilities within this organization learned a great deal by treating leishmaniasis in ways other than those recommended by MinSalud. This knowledge and skill set create valuable opportunities to work with ex-combatants and involve them in multidisciplinary efforts to bring therapeutic treatment alternatives to rural and remote areas in Colombia. I believe such a project presents an important opening for peace building.

Third, I believe there are at least two ways to change soldiers' experience with leishmaniasis to reduce harm. For one, the Army should offer education to its members so they can learn about what is known (and unknown) about the disease. This could help all military members understand the importance of evacuating soldiers from the war zone as soon as ulcers appear. It might also prevent the blaming and stigmatizing of soldiers when they become sick. Furthermore, Army personnel should receive public education materials not only on the disease but also on antileishmanial treatments, and they should be made aware of their rights if they have been affected by this disease. It is crucial to provide this information when young men first report to the Army to "define their military situation." In other words, the spread of ignorance and misinformation about leishmaniasis in the Army must be assertively challenged.

Finally, I believe that scientists are essential and powerful actors in achieving these goals. In my conversations with them during my fieldwork, I learned that they are frustrated because they believe there is a significant gap between their work and the changes needed to improve the lives of those impacted by leishmaniasis. For many, it is difficult to imagine how their work and position in society can contribute in meaningful ways to the creation of a nonviolent country. However, I believe that changing the relationship between war and leishmaniasis—starting with the actions just mentioned—depends to a great extent on laboratories and scientists. Scientists and their communities have more influence on public policy than a soldier or peasant. They should be able to examine their everyday practices to challenge the perpetration and perpetuation of violence that take place within biomedical research spaces. Moreover, their regular interactions with leishmaniasis patients from all over the country provide daily opportunities to understand other ways war and disease remain *enmarañados* and what can be done to produce alternative scenarios. At this pivotal point when peace building involves, even requires, individual and collective day-to-day commitments, scientific research projects must be carefully planned to earnestly and thoughtfully align the objectives of science with the objectives of peace.

Acknowledgments

In the many years it has taken to write, this book has come together through the support, kindness, sympathy, and encouragement that I was so fortunate to receive. Without the generosity of many individuals and institutions, this publication would not be in the hands of a reader intrigued by the lesser-known facets of the longest war endured by a Latin American nation.

I extend my heartfelt gratitude to the numerous Colombian Army soldiers, former guerrilla combatants, peasants, biomedical scientists, health care workers, public health officials, and kidnapping survivors who entrusted me with their stories and generously allowed me to gain profound insights into their lives.

I am immensely thankful to the Colombian Public Force, especially the military. Since my initial request for access to the Leishmaniasis Recovery Center (CRL), members of these institutions have consistently demonstrated sincere respect for my work. They have refrained from placing any requirements on the review of my research, allowing me total intellectual autonomy. It was a privilege to accompany both the soldier-patients and the military and civilian staff of the CRL through the vicissitudes of their daily routines.

I would also like to express my deep gratitude to the now-dissolved Revolutionary Armed Forces of Colombia guerrilla organization. I am humbled by all the ex-combatants committed to peace who gave me the opportunity to hear their experiences and to get closer to their past and present realities, and who found my research relevant to the challenging peace-building process still underway. I am honored to have had the chance to learn from such diverse perspectives and situations about the complexities of ending a protracted armed conflict amid hopes, promises, violence, and adversity.

I extend my gratitude to the Leishmaniasis Research Institute, the biomedical research facility I call LERI. Their tireless efforts to study leishmaniasis and provide health care to affected individuals in a remote area of Colombia have provided me with invaluable insights into the biomedical research of this disease within this particular context. Several people who are or have been affiliated with LERI were very generous in sharing their personal experiences and perspectives with me. Their help was pivotal in clarifying information and dispelling many of my uncertainties. Without institutions like LERI actively embracing interdisciplinary approaches and remaining open-minded to alternative viewpoints, conducting the necessary social and ethnographic research on topics entangled with scientific and technological dimensions would remain unrealized.

Generous financial support from York University and Manulife in Canada made my fieldwork possible. Funding from Colciencias, now the Colombian Ministry of Science, Technology and Innovation, was also essential to making this research a reality. Funding from the British Academy allowed me to devote time to writing this book as part of the "Diseased Landscapes" project. Institutional support from the Interdisciplinary Center for Development Studies at the Universidad de los Andes (Colombia), and in particular from Diana Ojeda, has been of tremendous importance to me, both academically and personally. Equally significant was the support of Javier Lezaun from the Institute for Science, Innovation and Society (InSIS) at the University of Oxford (UK). I am deeply grateful for the incredible privilege of working closely with both over the past few years. Thank you, Diana and Javier, for modeling a commitment to both rigorous and feminist academic practice, coupled with genuine care and empathy.

I would not have found the motivation to undertake this book project without the recognition I received from the Ann Johnson Institute for Science, Technology and Society at the University of South Carolina (US). Their award enabled me to workshop the manuscript and receive invaluable feedback from Ann Kelly, Ken MacLeish, Omar Dewachi, Magdalena Stawkowski, and Monica Barra. I cannot thank them enough, as well as Leah McClimans, Allison Marsh, and Emily Mathias for their efforts to make such a wonderful exchange possible despite the constraints imposed by the COVID-19 pandemic. I am also deeply grateful to the University of Chicago Press, especially Karen Darling, my editor, and Fabiola Enríquez, for their contributions to the editing and production of the book. Their dedication and hard work, alongside that of two anonymous reviewers, have been instrumental in making this publication possible and improving its quality.

Since the beginning of this research project, Denielle Elliott has provided me with invaluable mentorship and unwavering enthusiasm. I feel incredibly fortunate to have been able to rely on her insightful vision and guidance throughout. The quality of this work has also been greatly enhanced by the rigorous and thoughtful feedback of Alex Nading, Eric Mykhalovskiy, Deborah Neill, and Carlota McAllister. Tara Mahfoud and Daniel Ruiz Serna, valued friends rather than mere colleagues, generously devoted their time to reviewing the initial version of this manuscript. Their helpful comments and words of encouragement have spurred subsequent iterations, and Tara's companionship throughout the writing process has been a major source of inspiration and support. The painstaking task of meticulously refining the English language was undertaken by Denia Djokic. I am deeply grateful for her careful attention to detail and her equally thoughtful way of being a colleague and a friend.

I had several helpful conversations and received constructive feedback from a variety of people at different events, settings, and institutions. These include the School of Anthropology and Museum Ethnography at the University of Oxford (UK); the British Society for Parasitology (UK); the Political Entomologies seminar series, organized by the University of Cambridge (UK) and the Freie Universität Berlin (Germany); the Seminar of the Social and Economic Sciences Faculty at the Universidad del Valle (Colombia); the Program on Science, Technology, and Society at Harvard University (US); the Seminar of the History of Medicine Working Group at Harvard University (US); the Seminar of the Group of Social Studies of Illegality (GESI) at the Universidad Nacional (Colombia); the Seminar of the Research Group on Social Studies of Sciences, Technologies and Professions (GESCTP) at the Universidad del Rosario (Colombia); the Technoscience Salon organized by the University of Toronto and York University (Canada); the Doctoral School of Political and Social Studies of Science and Technology, organized by the Latin American Association of Social Studies of Science and Technology, ESOCITE; the National Colloquium of Social Studies of Science and Technology at the Universidad Nacional (Colombia); the Feminist Perspectives on Science and Technology Colloquium at the Universidad de los Andes (Colombia); the Centre for Imaginative Ethnography (Canada); and the Ethnographic Transdisciplinary Engagements Roundtable organized by the Science & Justice Research Center and Feminist Studies Department at the University of California, Santa Cruz (US).

Many networks, colleagues, and friends have offered their support in diverse ways throughout this journey. I would like to thank María Fernanda

Olarte, Tania Pérez Bustos, Diana Pardo Pedraza, Tatiana Acevedo, Nathalia Hernández, Adela Parra, Emma Shaw, Mady Barbeitas, Juan Pablo Centeno, Gabriel Ruiz, Simón Uribe, Stefan Pohl, Kristina Lyons, Juana Callejas, and Gwen Burnyeat for their support at various stages of this research and writing project. The meaningful friendship of Marcelo Aráus, Ana Carulla, David Ramírez, Serena Naim, María Adelaida Gómez, and Nicolás Sánchez also proved crucial. I am also grateful for the anticipatory musical celebrations with my dear neighbors Adriana Vásquez and Carlos Taboada, which always provide moments of joy and respite.

Finally, this book would not have come to fruition as a tangible object to be seen, touched, and perused without the unwavering and affectionate support of those nearest and dearest to my heart. I would like to express my deepest gratitude to Clemencia García, Juan Alfredo Pinto, María Elisa Pinto, Diego Junca, Alba Sáchica, and Juan Nieto. However, it is my life partner and steadfast reader, Diego Nieto, who deserves the utmost appreciation. None of this would have been possible without his companionship, relentless enthusiasm, and daily demonstrations of love. As I delved into crafting *Maraña*, Lorenzo joyously became part of our lives. Reflecting on how we navigated it all, I am filled with immense happiness seeing both the little human and the book inhabiting the world.

Notes

Introduction

1. Unless otherwise indicated, all the names used in this book are pseudonyms. I have altered some identifying details to ensure confidentiality.

2. In 2019, the Colombian anthropology journal *Maguaré* published a special issue titled *Conflict and Peace in Colombia Beyond the Human.* See Lyons, Pinto-García, and Ruiz Serna 2019.

3. A notable exception is a book in Portuguese, titled *Uma história das leishmanioses no novo mundo: fins do século XIX aos anos 1960*, edited by Jaime Benchimol and Denis Guedes Jogas Junior (2020), which deals with the history of leishmaniasis from a contextual perspective, with the main focus on Brazil.

4. In 1991, *Leishmania colombiensis* was described as a new parasite species, based on samples taken from humans, sandflies, and a sloth in Colombia and Panama (Kreutzer et al. 1991). Despite its name, this species is not the most widespread in the country. From the nine *Leishmania* parasite species that circulate in Colombia, *L. panamensis*, *L. braziliensis*, and *L. guyanensis* are most frequently involved in leishmaniasis cases (Ovalle-Bracho et al. 2019).

5. For example, Anderson 2006, 2008; Brown et al. 2006; Cueto 2006; Fassin 2012; Lezaun and Montgomery 2015; Neill 2012; Packard 2016; Quevedo et al. 2004; Stepan 2015.

6. See, for example, Ashford (2000), Choi and Lerner 2001, Dujardin et al. 2008, Pavli and Maltezou 2010, and Saravia and Nicholls 2006.

7. On the pharmaceuticalization of public health in developing countries, see also Whitmarsh 2008; Hayden 2007; S. E. Bell and Figert 2012.

8. The limited existing bibliography on the relationship between health and conflict in Colombia encompasses work exploring the injuries and disabilities caused by the war on the bodies of hundreds of thousands of combatants and civilians (Carmona Lozano 2016; CNMH and Fundación Prolongar 2017; Cohen 2012; Valencia et al. 2015). Important research has been developed on the effects of the ongoing armed violence on the mental health of civilians, especially on victims of forced internal displacement (Tamayo-Agudelo and Bell 2019; Gómez-Restrepo et al. 2016; V. Bell et al. 2012). Others have looked into the ways in which war sustains the structural violence that makes some people live in conditions of vulnerability to illness (Abadía and Oviedo 2009; Abadía et al. 2008; Cardona et al. 2005; Franco Agudelo 2003; Moreno and López

2009). Other research explores the destruction of health care infrastructures, the diversion of funds from health care to warfare, the disruption of the health system as a consequence of war, or violent actions against health care workers (Beyrer et al. 2007; Franco et al. 2006; D. Z. Urrego Mendoza 2003; Z. Urrego Mendoza 2011, 2015).

9. The association between war and health crises has been well established in many different contexts for a wide variety of diseases. See, for instance, Pedersen 2002; Ghobarah, Huth, and Russett 2004; Smallman-Raynor 2004; Levy and Sidel 2007; Berrang-Ford, Lundine, and Breau 2011; Ostrach and Singer 2012; R. Seaman 2018.

10. In 1935, Hans Zinsser (2010) published a highly popular biography of typhus, arguing that infectious diseases, and especially vector-borne typhus, have been far more decisive in the outcome of wars throughout history than humans and their military maneuvers. Andrew McIlwaine Bell (2010), Mariola Espinosa (2009), and Timothy Winegard (2019) have shown how mosquitoes have changed the course of various war events throughout history. Jeffrey Lockwood (2010) provides a historical overview of the weaponization of insects at different historical moments and, on that basis, discusses the present and future of entomological warfare.

11. See, for example, Dewachi 2015; Dewachi et al. 2014; Fassin 2009; Renne 2014; Westerhaus 2007. A rich and stimulating body of scholarship that understands illnesses as embodied experiences of violence has also been produced. See Adams 1998; Coker 2004; Fassin 2007; Green 1994; Henry 2006; Quesada 1998.

12. Very insightful scholarship taking a nonethnographic approach to exploring the conjunction of (bio)medicine and war has been produced. See J. Anderson and Perry 2014; Cooter 1993; Mark Harrison and Yim 2017; Linker 2011; Perry 2014.

13. Tragically, the number of victims of the Colombian armed conflict continues to grow. The figure of 9.5 million victims, which corresponds to approximately 19 percent of the Colombian population (fifty million people), was reported by the National Registrar of Victims (RUV), as of August 31, 2023 (https://www.unidadvictimas.gov.co/es/registro-unico-de-victimas-ruv/37394). This number corresponds to people who have been registered by the state as victimized in the scope of events related to the armed conflict, such as forced land abandonment or dispossession, terrorist actions, attacks, combats, threats, confinement, crimes against freedom and sexual integrity, forced disappearance, forced displacement, homicide, physical injuries, psychological injuries, antipersonnel mines, explosive devices, kidnapping, torture, recruitment of children and adolescents. For an STS exploration of the politics and practices involved in the construction of the RUV, see Mora-Gámez 2023.

14. See, for instance, Guarnizo Alvarez 2010; Molano Bravo 2005.

15. See, for example, *El Tiempo* 2008; Vélez and Pérez 2016. I come back to this in chapter 2.

Chapter One

1. See, for example, journalistic (Acevedo Serna 2012; *Contexto Ganadero* 2014; Minuto 2013, 30; Molano Bravo 2005b), scientific (Beyrer et al. 2007; PECET 2015; Velez et al. 2001; Zuleta and Velez 2014), and testimonial (Emanuelsson 2012; *Semana*, n.d.) accounts that have framed leishmaniasis as "the guerrilla disease."

2. This term, which seeks to hybridize *Fidel Castro* and *Hugo Chávez* in a fearsome communist chimera, was coined by former president Álvaro Uribe during his campaign against the peace negotiations and the agreement reached between the FARC and the government of Juan

Manuel Santos. Since then, it has been repeatedly used by him and others as an iterative slogan to discredit all sorts of people, actions, and opinions (see González 2017).

3. Burning wood that does not produce smoke is a strategic move because it avoids the aerial detection of guerrilla camps by the state Army.

4. Besides the article by Valderrama-Ardila et al. (2010) that I already mentioned, there are a few exceptions, such as the papers by Mónica Zuleta and Iván Darío Vélez (2014) and Patino et al. (2017).

5. The leishmaniasis case surveillance report form that the state uses is available here: https://www.ins.gov.co/buscador/Lineamientos/420_430_440_Leishmaniasis_2019.pdf.

6. In recent years, statisticians have pleaded for the embracement of uncertainty in science and the abandonment of the "statistically significant" terminology, based on the rigid rule of rejecting *p* values above 0.05 (see Oransky 2019). An editorial in a special issue of the American Statistician published in March 2019 offers an enlightening and refreshing perspective on this regard. "As we venture down this path," the editorial says, "we will begin to see fewer false alarms, fewer overlooked discoveries, and the development of more customized statistical strategies. Researchers will be free to communicate all their findings in all their glorious uncertainty, knowing their work is to be judged by the quality and effective communication of their science, and not by their *p*-values" (Wasserstein, Schirm, and Lazar 2019, 1).

Chapter Two

1. In 2017, 13,049 ex-FARC combatants initiated the reintegration process into civilian life (Fundación Ideas para la Paz and Oficina del Alto Comisionado para la Paz 2019).

2. According to MinSalud's clinical practice guideline, Glucantime therapy involves a once-a-day administration of 2 injections, given in the buttocks over 20 days (28 days in the case of mucosal leishmaniasis). Not every patient receives the same volume of Glucantime because the daily dose is calculated based on the patient's weight: 20 mg of antimony per kilogram. For heavier patients, however, the administration of the drug cannot be higher than 4 ampoules per day (20 ml of Glucantime). In those cases, MinSalud (2018) recommends increasing the number of days to complete the overall dose. To give an example of how many ampoules of Glucantime an adult would need, let's assume that a female patient weighs 70 kg. She would daily require 17.29 ml of Glucantime divided in 2 injections, which corresponds to 69.16 ampoules, each one containing 5 ml of the drug. Once a vial has been opened, however, the remnants should not be saved for the next day. Thus, 17.29 ml of Glucantime require the use of 4 ampoules a day, that is, 80 ampoules for 20 days of treatment.

3. Meta is a *departamento* located in the center-east of the country.

4. See Danish Institute for International Studies 2009, 16n20. I am indebted to Daniel Ruiz-Serna for pointing this out.

5. *Secretarías departamentales de salud* and *secretarías distritales de salud.*

6. These facilities are officially known in Colombia as *Instituciones Prestadoras de Servicios de Salud*, or IPSs.

7. In the case of antibiotics, for example, existing legislation establishes that their sale is prohibited without a medical prescription since 2005. However, the enforcement of these norms has been restricted to Bogotá. As Vacca et al. (2011) showed in a study using undercover care seekers, most pharmacies in Bogotá (80.3 percent of 239 pharmacies involved in the study) required no prescription to sell these drugs.

8. Although it is misleading and unethical to fuse into one entity civilians and members of guerrilla and paramilitary groups, this slippage in language reflects how these two populations are hardly discernable in a guerrilla warfare and get easily and dangerously conflated.

9. For an analysis of the emergence and the implications of WHO's global public health security framework, see Lakoff 2017.

10. Biomedical research institutions conducting studies on leishmaniasis, whose clinical facilities are officially constituted as IPSs, are an exception to this rule.

11. In Spanish, *seguridad* means both "security" and "safety."

12. The values in US dollars are calculated based on the average exchange rate in 2016, equivalent to 3050.98 Colombian pesos for one US dollar (see http://www.banrep.gov.co/es/estadisticas/trm).

13. For Colombians, these stories of corruption are outrageous but not surprising. Corruption is perceived as one of the most pressing, deep-rooted, and widespread problems in Colombia (Gallup Colombia 2017; Henao and Isaza 2018). In 2021, Transparency International published an analysis of acts of corruption in Colombia that were reported in twenty-five media outlets between 2016 and 2020. It concluded that the Army and the Police are among the most corrupt state entities (*El Espectador* 2021).

14. See also US Embassy in Colombia 2005d.

15. See, for instance, *El Tiempo* 2006, 2008, 2009b, 2009c, 2009a; MOE and Fundación Ciudad Abierta 2017; RCN Radio 2015; Monsalve Gaviria 2017.

16. See, for example, AFP 2013; Areacucuta 2013; Canal Uno 2011; Diario del Huila 2011; *El Colombiano* 2005; *El Espectador* 2014; Llanera 2011; Territorio Chocoano 2011; Vanguardia 2014.

17. Before becoming a political party in 2016, the FARC was headed by a commander in chief, followed by a group of seven male guerrilla leaders called the FARC Secretariat.

18. See *Contexto Ganadero* 2014; *El Nuevo Siglo* 2011; *El Tiempo* 2001; *La Patria* 2013; *Semana* 2015; Guarnizo Alvarez 2010; Acevedo Serna 2012.

Chapter Three

1. Throughout the twenty days of Glucantime treatment, leishmaniasis patients lose several kilograms of weight. Unlike other places, in the Army, the dose is adjusted daily according to weight loss. If this is not done, patients may be overdosed.

2. The following men may be exempted from compulsory military service: persons with permanent physical and sensory disabilities, Indigenous people residing in their territory, victims of the internal armed conflict, demobilized people, single children, clergy and religious persons, married persons sentenced to penalties, siblings or children of persons who have died or acquired an absolute and permanent disability as a member of the Public Force, children of parents unable to work or over sixty years of age, and orphans of parents if they financially support their siblings (Ámbito Jurídico 2015).

3. Although to a lesser extent, secondary school graduates may also be recruited by the Police as *auxiliar de policía bachiller* (secondary school graduate police assistant).

4. One of those valuable initiatives is the Collective Action of Conscientious Objectors. See https://www.facebook.com/objetoresyobjetorasdeconciencia/

5. A few majors enter the area of operations when they are commanders within counterinsurgency battalions.

6. Data from the Directorate for Integral Action Against Antipersonnel Mines (DAICMA) database available here: http://www.accioncontraminas.gov.co/estadisticas/Paginas/Bases-de-Datos.aspx. These figures include mortal and nonmortal victims of both land mines and unexploded ordnance.

7. Urabá is a region in northwestern Colombia with a strong presence of armed actors since the 1970s and has experienced significant violence related to the armed conflict since the mid-1990s.

8. "Casualty" refers to the withdrawal of combatants from military duties due to death, injury, illness, capture, or desertion. Any soldier who is killed, injured, sick, or hospitalized is a casualty. Although the word is commonly used synonymously with *fatality*, nonfatal injuries and disease also lead to military casualties.

9. These figures, kindly provided by the Army upon my request, include both cases of cutaneous (98.2%) and mucosal leishmaniasis (1.8%). However, the actual number of servicemen with leishmaniasis is difficult to determine, as some soldiers were infected more than once. Thus, some individuals have been counted more than once.

10. The Public Force uses a typology to classify psychophysical lesions and determine the associated institutional obligations and compensations. This typology, enforced by the Decree 1796 of 2000 (https://www.sanidadfuerzasmilitares.mil.co/english/the_entity/normativity/decrees/decreto_1796_2000), is known among the military as "*los literales*," which correspond to four types of circumstances under which psychophysical lesions may occur:

Literal A: In the service, but not for cause and reason thereof; that is, illness and/or common accident.

Literal B: In the service, for cause and reason thereof; that is, occupational disease and/or workplace accident.

Literal C: In the service, as a result of combat or in an accident related to it, or by direct action of the enemy, in tasks of maintenance or restoration of public order, or in international conflict.

Literal D: In acts carried out against the law, the regulation, or the superior order.

Thus, leishmaniasis is considered a *Literal B* type of lesion.

11. As I describe in chapter 2, a Ministry of Health officer told me that in the past, "of every six [leishmaniasis] patients, five medications were in the Army and one in the civilian population." In an access to information request, I asked the Ministry of Health to provide data of Glucantime distribution since the 1940s. The ministry claimed to have data only from 2010 onward, so I received data only from 2010 until 2018. Nevertheless, I was able to corroborate that, in 2010, when 38 percent of the leishmaniasis cases in Colombia were reported by the military, the Army received 71.6 percent of the Glucantime ampoules the state had purchased in that year. With the exception of 2012, in all subsequent years, civilians have been given more than 50 percent of the Glucantime acquired.

12. The average ampoule price between 1997 and 2007 was COP 6,266 (about USD 2). The average ampoule price since the participation of the Colombian state in the PAHO Strategic Fund until 2017 was COP 2,618 (approximately USD 0.8). Thus, the ampoule price has decreased in by 58.2 percent in twenty years. These calculations are based on data provided by the Ministry of Health through an access to information request.

13. Nopikex is the main product manufactured by the small Colombian company Salder Limitada, which is dedicated to the production of repellents. In contrast, Ultrathon is produced by 3M, formerly known as the Minnesota Mining and Manufacturing Company, a large

multinational American company with operations in more than seventy countries. 3M manufactures a wide variety of products, Scotch Tape being the best known.

14. In 2014, miltefosine became the first and only drug approved by the US Food and Drug Administration for the treatment of cutaneous leishmaniasis.

15. At the time of my fieldwork (2017), there were only four military dermatologists in the Army.

16. Male nursing assistants only undertook these responsibilities on the weekends.

Chapter Four

1. The impact of both leishmaniasis and antileishmanial drugs on fertility is a very under-researched area of study. According to Coelho et al. (2014, 98): "The safety of [pentavalent antimonials like Glucantime] was not thoroughly evaluated prior to their introduction into clinical practice in the mid-1940s, and since then, major gaps in their safety profile have remained unfilled. One of these gaps in the toxicity data for [pentavalent antimonials] is the lack of preclinical studies on the reproductive toxicity and kinetics during pregnancy and lactation." Nonetheless, the Colombian Army does recognize the loss of fertility as a consequence of leishmaniasis treatments and pays compensation to soldiers who have undergone antileishmanial therapy and who medically demonstrate, through a spermogram, deficiencies in their reproductive ability.

2. In Latin America, the efficacy of pentavalent antimonials like Glucantime is 76.5% (Tuon et al. 2008).

3. Soldiers frequently complained that despite these recommendations, the refreshments they received at the CRL often included Coca-Cola.

4. Glucantime is harmful to the heart. Therefore, it is important for patients not to exert too much stress on this vital organ. Nonetheless, in military clinical settings other than the CRL, soldiers are not exempt from labor and physical activities.

5. It was said that vitamins strengthened the *Leishmania* parasites more than the soldier's body.

6. Throughout the treatment, soldiers are often told not to have any sexual activity and not to take any psychoactive drugs.

7. See Decree 1796 of 2000, available at https://www.sanidadfuerzasmilitares.mil.co/english/the_entity/normativity/decrees/decreto_1796_2000.

8. The economic compensation is calculated based on a classification and score system established by the Decree 0094 of 1989 (available at https://www.sanidadfuerzasmilitares.mil.co/english/the_entity/normativity/decrees/decreto_94_1989). Leishmaniasis scars on the face, for example, have a higher score—involve a higher compensation—than leishmaniasis scars located on other parts of the body.

9. Interestingly, scientists who study leishmaniasis like to call themselves *leishmaniacs*—the English version of *leishmaníacos*.

10. One scientific article states that out of a sample of 221 soldiers with leishmaniasis, 31 percent had contracted it at least once (Patino et al. 2017).

Chapter Five

1. In December 2019, Colciencias became the Ministry of Science, Technology and Innovation (MinCiencias).

2. Research on leishmaniasis has gained momentum thanks to a group of high-profile scientists, most of them partially trained in North America and Europe. In the 1980s, they identified leishmaniasis as an underexplored research topic at both the national and international levels. World-renowned institutions such as the International Center for Medical Research and Training (CIDEIM) and the Program for the Study and Control of Tropical Diseases at the University of Antioquia (PECET) are the most representative examples of this trajectory. Currently, many of the scientists who conduct research not only on leishmaniasis but also other infectious diseases in various universities and scientific institutions in Colombia were trained in the laboratories of CIDEIM and PECET.

3. See, for instance, Contreras et al., 2012; Ocampo et al., 2012; Pardo et al., 2006; Santaella et al., 2011; Valderrama-Ardila et al., 2010; Vega et al., 2007, 2009.

4. As I explained in chapter 1, scientists were surprised by the sudden emergence of leishmaniasis in Chaparral. Before 2003, leishmaniasis was very rare in that area.

5. Many soldiers recovering from leishmaniasis at the CRL told me they thought it was guerrillas who somehow released leishmaniasis in the jungle to harm state troops. And many guerrillas told me they believed it was the state that had devised a sort of leishmaniasis bioweapon to affect subversive groups. Although leishmaniasis is a pre-Hispanic disease that even ceramists of the Moche culture (100–700 AD) carved on human figures well before the Spanish set a foot on these lands (Altamirano-Enciso et al. 2003), war logic has made it plausible to think of leishmaniasis as a sort of recently introduced biological weapon.

6. In Colombia, people conventionally refer to the smear procedure through which cutaneous leishmaniasis is typically diagnosed as *raspado* (scraping).

References

Aagaard-Hansen, Jens, Nohelly Nombela, and Jorge Alvar. 2010. "Population Movement: A Key Factor in the Epidemiology of Neglected Tropical Diseases: Population Movement and Neglected Tropical Diseases." *Tropical Medicine & International Health* 15 (11): 1281–88. https://doi.org/10.1111/j.1365-3156.2010.02629.x.

Abadía, César, Germán Cortés, E. Fino, C. García, D. Oviedo, and M. Y. Pinilla Alfonso. 2008. "Perspectivas Inter-Situadas Sobre El Capitalismo En La Salud: Desde Colombia y Sobre Colombia." *Palimpsestus* 6:163–76.

Abadía, César Ernesto, and Diana G. Oviedo. 2009. "Bureaucratic Itineraries in Colombia. A Theoretical and Methodological Tool to Assess Managed-Care Health Care Systems." *Social Science & Medicine* 68 (6): 1153–60. https://doi.org/10.1016/j.socscimed.2008.12.049.

Abraham, John. 2010. "Pharmaceuticalization of Society in Context: Theoretical, Empirical and Health Dimensions." *Sociology* 44 (4): 603–22. https://doi.org/10.1177/0038038510369368.

Acevedo Serna, Natalia. 2012. "Leishmaniasis, ¿una Marca de La Guerra?" *Infrarrojo*. Teleantioquia. https://www.youtube.com/watch?v=570g9D9JKXY.

Adams, Vincanne. 1998. "Suffering the Winds of Lhasa: Politicized Bodies, Human Rights, Cultural Difference, and Humanism in Tibet." *Medical Anthropology Quarterly* 12 (1): 74–102.

Adams-Hutcheson, Gail. 2017. "Spatialising Skin: Pushing the Boundaries of Trauma Geographies." *Emotion, Space and Society*, 24 (August): 105–12. https://doi.org/10.1016/j.emospa.2016.03.002.

AFP. 2013. "Decomisan Medicina Contra La Leishmaniasis Supuestamente Para La Guerrilla." *El Espectador*, November 20, 2013. http://www.elespectador.com/noticias/judicial/decomisan-medicina-contra-leishmaniasis-supuestamente-g-articulo-459516.

Ahmed, Sara, and Jackie Stacey. 2001. *Thinking Through the Skin*. New York: Routledge.

Alawieh, Ali, Umayya Musharrafieh, Amani Jaber, Atika Berry, Nada Ghosn, and Abdul Rahman Bizri. 2014. "Revisiting Leishmaniasis in the Time of War: The Syrian Conflict and the Lebanese Outbreak." *International Journal of Infectious Diseases* 29 (December): 115–19. https://doi.org/10.1016/j.ijid.2014.04.023.

Altamirano-Enciso, Alfredo J., Mauro C. A. Marzochi, João S. Moreira, Armando O. Schubach, and Keyla B. F. Marzochi. 2003. "On the Origin and Spread of Cutaneous and Mucosal

Leishmaniasis, Based on Pre-and Post-Colombian Historical Sources." *História, Ciências, Saúde-Manguinhos* 10 (3): 853–82.

Alvar, Jorge, Iván D. Vélez, Caryn Bern, Mercé Herrero, Philippe Desjeux, Jorge Cano, Jean Jannin, Margriet den Boer, and the WHO Leishmaniasis Control Team. 2012. "Leishmaniasis Worldwide and Global Estimates of Its Incidence." *PLoS ONE* 7 (5): e35671. https://doi.org/10.1371/journal.pone.0035671.

Ámbito Jurídico. 2015. "Estas son las personas eximidas del servicio militar." Legis Ámbito Jurídico. June 12, 2015. https://www.ambitojuridico.com/noticias/general/administrativo-y-contratacion/estas-son-las-personas-eximidas-del-servicio-militar.

Anderson, Julie, and Heather R. Perry. 2014. "Rehabilitation and Restoration: Orthopaedics and Disabled Soldiers in Germany and Britain in the First World War." *Medicine, Conflict and Survival* 30 (4): 227–51. https://doi.org/10.1080/13623699.2014.962724.

Anderson, Warwick. 2006. *Colonial Pathologies: American Tropical Medicine, Race, and Hygiene in the Philippines*. Durham, NC: Duke University Press.

———. 2008. *The Collectors of Lost Souls: Turning Kuru Scientists into Whitemen*. Baltimore: Johns Hopkins University Press.

Andreas, Peter. 2020. *Killer High: A History of War in Six Drugs*. Oxford: Oxford University Press.

Angarita, Pablo Emilio. 2011. *Seguridad Democrática: Lo Invisible de Un Régimen Político y Económico*. Bogotá: Siglo del Hombre Editores.

Areacucuta. 2013. "Incautado alijo de 625 ampollas de Glucantime para el tratamiento de la Leishmaniasis visceral y cutánea." *Areacucuta*, November 20, 2013. https://www.areacucuta.com/incautado-alijo-de-625-ampollas-de-glucantime-para-el-tratamiento-de-la-leishmaniasis-visceral-y-cutanea/.

Arjona, Ana. 2016. *Rebelocracy: Social Order in the Colombian Civil War*. New York: Cambridge University Press.

Arteta, Carolina. 2018. "Ir al médico, toda una odisea en la Colombia rural." *Semana Rural*, May 22, 2018. https://semanarural.com/articulo/ir-al-medico-toda-una-odisea-en-la-colombia-rural/527.

Ashford, R. W. 2000. "The Leishmaniases as Emerging and Reemerging Zoonoses." *International Journal for Parasitology* 30 (12): 1269–81.

Avendaño Ladino, Laura María. 2023. "Habrá homenaje en Bogotá a líderes y excombatientes asesinados tras el Acuerdo de Paz." *El Tiempo*, August 18, 2023, sec. bogota. https://www.eltiempo.com/bogota/invitan-a-homenaje-a-lideres-sociales-y-firmantes-de-paz-asesinados-797444.

Ávila, Ariel. 2019. *Detrás de La Guerra En Colombia*. Bogotá: Planeta.

Ávila Guarnizo, Leonid. 2010. "Letter from Attorney Leonid A. Guarnizo to the 10th Attorney in the Unit for Human Rights and International Humanitarian Law, Regarding the Process about the Enforced Disappearance, Torture and Murder of Simón Efraín González Ramírez," August 2, 2010. *Verdad Abierta*.

Baader, Gerhard, Susan E. Lederer, Morris Low, Florian Schmaltz, and Alexander V. Schwerin. 2005. "Pathways to Human Experimentation, 1933–1945: Germany, Japan, and the United States." *Osiris* 20:205–31.

Barbeitas, Mady. 2019. "The Innovation System for Leishmaniasis Therapy in Brazil." In *Health Innovation and Social Justice in Brazil*, edited by Maurice Cassier and Marilena Correa, 109–34. Cham: Palgrave Macmillan. https://doi.org/10.1007/978-3-319-76834-2.

———. 2020. "L'écosystème de l'innovation—Des Enjeux Scientifiques, Économiques et Politiques Sur Les Leishmanioses." PhD diss., École des Hautes Études en Sciences Sociales (EHESS).

Barreto-Romero, Juan David, María Alejandra Ortíz-Forero, and Cristian Danilo Cely. 2020. "Revisión histórica de la incorporación y participación de la mujer en el arma de Infantería del Ejército Nacional de Colombia." *Estudios en Seguridad y Defensa* 15 (30): 373–92. https://doi.org/10.25062/1900-8325.267.

Bedoya Lima, Jineth. 2006a. "William, Dos Años Metido En Las Selvas Del Patriota." *El Tiempo*, May 7, 2006. http://www.eltiempo.com/archivo/documento/MAM-2013908.

———. 2006b. "Fin Del Plan Patriota, Llega El Plan Victoria." *El Tiempo*, December 10, 2006. http://www.eltiempo.com/archivo/documento/MAM-2312800.

Beiter, Kaylin J., Zachariah J. Wentlent, Adrian R. Hamouda, and Bolaji N. Thomas. 2019. "Nonconventional Opponents: A Review of Malaria and Leishmaniasis among United States Armed Forces." *PeerJ* 7 (January). https://doi.org/10.7717/peerj.6313.

Bell, Andrew McIlwaine. 2010. *Mosquito Soldiers: Malaria, Yellow Fever, and the Course of the American Civil War*. Baton Rouge: Louisiana State University Press.

Bell, Susan E., and Anne E. Figert. 2012. "Medicalization and Pharmaceuticalization at the Intersections: Looking Backward, Sideways and Forward." *Social Science & Medicine (1982)* 75 (5): 775–83. https://doi.org/10.1016/j.socscimed.2012.04.002.

Bell, Vaughan, Fernanda Méndez, Carmen Martínez, Pedro Pablo Palma, and Marc Bosch. 2012. "Characteristics of the Colombian Armed Conflict and the Mental Health of Civilians Living in Active Conflict Zones." *Conflict and Health* 6 (1): 10. https://doi.org/10.1186/1752-1505-6-10.

Benchimol, Jaime Larry, Frederico da Costa Gualandi, Danielle Cristina dos Santos Barreto, and Luciana de Araujo Pinheiro. 2019. "Leishmaniasis: Historical Configuration in Brazil with an Emphasis on the Visceral Disease, from the 1930s to the 1960s." *Boletim Do Museu Paraense Emílio Goeldi. Ciências Humanas* 14 (2): 611–26. https://doi.org/10.1590/1981.81222019000200017.

Benchimol, Jaime Larry, and Denis Guedes Jogas Junior. 2020. *Uma História Das Leishmanioses No Novo Mundo: Fins Do Século XIX Aos Anos 1960*. Rio de Janeiro: Fiocruz.

Berrang-Ford, Lea, Jamie Lundine, and Sebastien Breau. 2011. "Conflict and Human African Trypanosomiasis." *Social Science & Medicine* 72 (3): 398–407. https://doi.org/10.1016/j.socscimed.2010.06.006.

Berry, Isha, and Lea Berrang-Ford. 2016. "Leishmaniasis, Conflict, and Political Terror: A Spatio-Temporal Analysis." *Social Science & Medicine (1982)*, May. https://doi.org/10.1016/j.socscimed.2016.04.038.

Betancourt, Ingrid. 2010. *Even Silence Has an End: My Six Years of Captivity in the Colombian Jungle*. New York: Penguin.

Beyrer, Chris, Juan Carlos Villar, Voravit Suwanvanichkij, Sonal Singh, Stefan D. Baral, and Edward J. Mills. 2007. "Neglected Diseases, Civil Conflicts, and the Right to Health." *Lancet* 370 (9587): 619–27.

Bickford, Andrew. 2020. *Chemical Heroes: Pharmacological Supersoldiers in the US Military*. Durham, NC: Duke University Press.

Biehl, João. 2007. *Will to Live: AIDS Therapies and the Politics of Survival*. Princeton, NJ: Princeton University Press.

Bijker, Wiebe E., and John Law, eds. 1994. *Shaping Technology / Building Society: Studies in Sociotechnical Change*. Cambridge, MA: MIT Press.

Birn, Anne-Emanuelle. 2005. "Gates's Grandest Challenge: Transcending Technology as Public Health Ideology." *Lancet* 366 (9484): 514–19. https://doi.org/10.1016/S0140-6736(05)66479-3.

Blair Trujillo, Elsa. 2009. "Aproximación Teórica al Concepto de Violencia: Avatares de una Definición." *Política y Cultura*, no. 32, 9–33.

Bowker, Geoffrey C., and Susan Leigh Star. 1999. *Sorting Things Out: Classification and Its Consequences*. Cambridge, MA: MIT Press.

Braveman, Paula, and Laura Gottlieb. 2014. "The Social Determinants of Health: It's Time to Consider the Causes of the Causes." *Public Health Reports* 129 (Suppl. 2): 19–31.

Brown, Hannah, and Ann H. Kelly. 2014. "Material Proximities and Hotspots: Toward an Anthropology of Viral Hemorrhagic Fevers." *Medical Anthropology Quarterly* 28 (2): 280–303. https://doi.org/10.1111/maq.12092.

Brown, Theodore, Marcos Cueto, and Elizabeth Fee. 2006. "The World Health Organization and the Transition from 'International' to 'Global' Public Health." *American Journal of Public Health* 96 (1): 62–72.

Camargo, Alejandro, and Diana Ojeda. 2017. "Ambivalent Desires: State Formation and Dispossession in the Face of Climate Crisis." *Political Geography* 60 (September): 57–65. https://doi.org/10.1016/j.polgeo.2017.04.003.

Canal Uno. 2011. "Contrabando de Glucantime Para Las FARC." *Canal Uno*, November 13, 2011. https://canal1.com.co/noticias/contrabando-de-glucantime-para-las-farc/.

Cárdenas, Carlos, and Carlos Arturo Duarte Torres. 2016. "Proxémica, Kinésica y Antropología. Apuntes Sobre Simulación Etnográfica, Cuerpo y Espacio En El Marco Del Conflicto Armado Colombiano." *Antipoda* 25 (May): 33–58. https://doi.org/10.7440/antipoda25.2016.02.

Cardona, Álvaro, O. Mejía, Luz Mery, L. Nieto, and V. Restrepo. 2005. "Temas Críticos En La Reforma de La Ley de Seguridad Social de Colombia En El Capítulo de Salud." *Revista Facultad Nacional de Salud Pública* 23 (1): 117–33.

Carmona Lozano, Mabel. 2016. "Entre El Amor y El Odio. Reflexiones En Torno al Trabajo de Campo Con Soldados Profesionales Del Ejército Colombiano." *Ecuador Debate* 99:103–17.

CEV. 2021. *La Guerra No Sana Heridas: Reconocimiento de Los Impactos Del Conflicto Armado Colombiano En La Salud*. Bogotá. https://web.comisiondelaverdad.co/actualidad/publicaciones/la-guerra-no-sana-heridas-2.

Choi, Christine M., and Ethan A. Lerner. 2001. "Leishmaniasis as an Emerging Infection." *Journal of Investigative Dermatology Symposium Proceedings* 6:175–82.

Chua, Jocelyn Lim. 2018. "Fog of War: Psychopharmaceutical 'Side Effects' and the United States Military." *Medical Anthropology* 37 (1): 17–31. https://doi.org/10.1080/01459740.2016.1235571.

CINEP. 2010. "Panorama de Derechos Humanos." *Noche y Niebla* 42. https://www.cinep.org.co/publicaciones/PDFS/20101201.nocheyniebla42.pdf.

Ciro Rodríguez, Estefanía. 2020. *Levantados de La Selva: Vidas y Legitimidades En Los Territorios Cocaleros*. Bogotá: Universidad de los Andes.

Clare, Eli. 2017. *Brilliant Imperfection: Grappling with Cure*. Durham, NC: Duke University Press.

CNMH. 2013. *¡Basta Ya! Colombia: Memorias de Guerra y Dignidad*. Bogotá: Centro Nacional de Memoria Histórica.

———. 2014. *Guerrilla y Población Civil: Trayectoria de Las FARC 1949 - 2013*. 3d ed. Bogotá: Centro Nacional de Memoria Histórica.

———. 2018. *Todo Pasó Frente a Nuestros Ojos. El Genocidio de La Unión Patriótica 1984-2002*. Bogotá: Centro Nacional de Memoria Histórica.

CNMH and Fundación Prolongar. 2017. *La Guerra Escondida: Minas Antipersonal y Remanentes Explosivos En Colombia*. Bogotá: Centro Nacional de Memoria Histórica.

Coelho, Deise R., Rosangela R. De-Carvalho, Rafael C. C. Rocha, Tatiana D. Saint'Pierre, and Francisco J. R. Paumgartten. 2014. "Effects of in Utero and Lactational Exposure to SbV on Rat Neurobehavioral Development and Fertility." *Reproductive Toxicology* 50 (December): 98–107. https://doi.org/10.1016/j.reprotox.2014.10.016.

Cohen, Emily. 2012. "From Phantoms to Prostheses." *Disability Studies Quarterly* 32 (3). http://dsq-sds.org/article/view/3269.

———. 2015. "Disciplining Pain: Masculinity and Ideologies of Repair in a Colombian Military Hospital." *Body & Society* 21 (3): 91–114. https://doi.org/10.1177/1357034X15586241.

Coker, Elizabeth Marie. 2004. "'Traveling Pains': Embodied Metaphors of Suffering among Southern Sudanese Refugees in Cairo." *Culture, Medicine and Psychiatry* 28 (1): 15–39.

Colombia2020. 2017. "La marcha final de las Farc hacia las zonas veredales." *El Espectador*, January 30, 2017. https://www.elespectador.com/colombia2020/territorio/la-marcha-final-de-las-farc-hacia-las-zonas-veredales-articulo-855126.

Conrad, Peter. 2005. "The Shifting Engines of Medicalization." *Journal of Health and Social Behavior* 46 (1): 3–14. https://doi.org/10.1177/002214650504600102.

Contexto Ganadero. 2014. "Medicina Contra Leishmaniasis La Nueva 'vacuna' de las Farc." *Contexto Ganadero*, September 30, 2014. http://www.contextoganadero.com/regiones/medicina-contra-leishmaniasis-la-nueva-vacuna-de-las-farc.

Contreras, María Angélica, Rafael José Vivero, Eduar Elías Bejarano, Lina María Carrillo, and Iván Darío Vélez. 2012. "New Records of Phlebotomine Sand Flies (Diptera: Psychodidae) Near the Amoya River in Chaparral, Tolima." *Biomedica* 32 (2): 263–68. https://doi.org/10.1590/S0120-41572012000300014.

Cooter, Roger. 1990. "Medicine and the Goodness of War." *Canadian Bulletin of Medical History* 7 (2): 147–59. https://doi.org/10.3138/cbmh.7.2.147.

———. 1993. *Surgery and Society in Peace and War: Orthopaedics and the Organization of Modern Medicine, 1880–1948*. London: Palgrave Macmillan.

Cooter, Roger, and Steve Sturdy. 1998. "Of War, Medicine and Modernity." In *War, Medicine and Modernity*, edited by Roger Cooter, Mark Harrison, and Steve Sturdy, 1–21. Gloucestershire: Sutton.

Correa-Cárdenas, Camilo A., Julie Pérez, Luz H. Patino, Juan David Ramírez, Maria Clara Duque, Yanira Romero, Omar Cantillo-Barraza, Omaira Rodríguez, María Teresa Alvarado, Claudia Cruz, and Claudia Méndez. 2020. "Distribution, Treatment Outcome and Genetic Diversity of Leishmania Species in Military Personnel from Colombia with Cutaneous Leishmaniasis." *BMC Infectious Diseases* 20 (1): 1–11. https://doi.org/10.1186/s12879-020-05529-y.

Crosby, Alfred W. 2003. *America's Forgotten Pandemic: The Influenza of 1918*. Cambridge: Cambridge University Press.

Cruz, Claudia. 2016. "Aspectos Clínicos, Epidemiológicos y Manejo de Pacientes Con Leishmaniasis En El Ejército de Colombia." In *Memorias 1ra Reunión Colombiana de Leishmaniasis y Chagas*, 8. Medellín. http://pecet-colombia.org/site/images/documentos/MemoriasReuni%C3%B3nSimposioPECET.pdf.

Cruz, Edwin. 2015. "Relaciones cívico-militares, negociaciones de paz y postconflicto en Colombia." *Criterio Jurídico Garantista* 8 (13): 12–41.

Cueto, Marcos. 2006. *The Value of Health: A History of the Pan American Health Organization.* Washington, DC: Pan American Health Organization.

Curtin, Philip D. 1989. *Death by Migration.* Cambridge: Cambridge University Press.

Danish Institute for International Studies. 2009. "Synthesis Report: Civil-Military Relations in International Operations." 16. Copenhagen. https://www.econstor.eu/bitstream/10419/59837/1/598756418.pdf.

Davis Marsden, Philip. 1985. "Pentavalent Antimonials: Old Drugs for New Diseases." *Revista Da Sociedade Brasileira de Medicina Tropical* 18 (3): 187–98.

De Abreu, Lissy. 2017. "Farc construyen poblado ecológico y sustentable para vivir en Colombia." *El Espectador*, June 17, 2017. https://www.elespectador.com/noticias/nacional/farc-construyen-poblado-ecologico-y-sustentable-para-vivir-en-colombia-articulo-698845.

Debus, Allen G. 2001. *Chemistry and Medical Debate: Van Helmont to Boerhaave.* Canton, MA: Watson.

Defensoría del Pueblo. 2014. "Servicio Militar Obligatorio en Colombia: Incorporación, Reclutamiento y Objeción de Conciencia." Bogotá. http://defensoria.gov.co/public/pdf/ServicioMilitarObligatorio.pdf.

De León, Jason. 2015. *The Land of Open Graves: Living and Dying on the Migrant Trail.* Oakland: University of California Press.

Dewachi, Omar. 2015. "When Wounds Travel." *Medicine Anthropology Theory* 2 (3): 61. https://doi.org/10.17157/mat.2.3.182.

———. 2017. *Ungovernable Life: Mandatory Medicine and Statecraft in Iraq.* Stanford: Stanford University Press.

———. 2019. "Iraqibacter and the Pathologies of Intervention." *Middle East Report*, July 2, 2019. https://merip.org/2019/07/iraqibacter-and-the-pathologies-of-intervention/.

Dewachi, Omar, Mac Skelton, Vinh-Kim Nguyen, Fouad M. Fouad, Ghassan Abu Sitta, Zeina Maasri, and Rita Giacaman. 2014. "Changing Therapeutic Geographies of the Iraqi and Syrian Wars." *Lancet* 383 (9915): 449–57. https://doi.org/10.1016/S0140-6736(13)62299-0.

DGSM. 2008. "Directiva No. 118 de 2018. Calificación En Primera Oportunidad de Las Contingencias de Origen Laboral."

Diario del Huila. 2011. "Incautados Medicamentos Con Destino a Las Farc." *Diario Del Huila*, November 14, 2011. http://www.ideaspaz.org/tools/download/60646.

Diaz, Ileana I., and Alison Mountz. 2020. "Intensifying Fissures: Geopolitics, Nationalism, Militarism, and the US Response to the Novel Coronavirus." *Geopolitics* 25 (5): 1037–44. https://doi.org/10.1080/14650045.2020.1789804.

Didwania, Nicky, Md Shadab, Abdus Sabur, and Nahid Ali. 2017. "Alternative to Chemotherapy—The Unmet Demand against Leishmaniasis." *Frontiers in Immunology* 8:1779. https://doi.org/10.3389/fimmu.2017.01779.

DNDi. 2023. "Cutaneous Leishmaniasis." DNDi. 2023. https://dndi.org/diseases/cutaneous-leishmaniasis/.

Duarte da Silva, Matheus Alves. 2023. "Between Deserts and Jungles: The Emergence and Circulation of Sylvatic Plague (1920–1950)." *Medical Anthropology* 42 (4): 1–15. https://doi.org/10.1080/01459740.2023.2189110.

Dujardin, Jean-Claude, Lenea Campino, Carmen Canavate, Jean-Pierre Dedet, Luigi Gradoni, Ketty Soteriadou, Apostolos Mazeris, Yusuf Ozbel, and Marleen Boelaert. 2008. "Spread of Vector-Borne Diseases and Neglect of Leishmaniasis, Europe." *Emerging Infectious Diseases* 14 (7).

Dumit, Joseph. 2012. *Drugs for Life. How Pharmaceutical Companies Define Our Health.* Durham, NC: Duke University Press.

Durand, M. M. P., M. Benmussa, and M. Caruana. 1946. "Traitment Du Kala-Azar Par Un Nouveau Composé Stibié: Le 2.168 R.P. (Premiers Résultats)." *Bulletins et Mémoires de La Société Medicale Des Hopitaux de Paris* 62 (24–25): 399–409.

Dutta, Achintya Kumar. 2008. "Pursuit of Medical Knowledge: Charles Donovan (1863–1951) on Kala-Azar in India." *Journal of Medical Biography* 16 (2): 72–76. https://doi.org/10.1258/jmb.2007.007004.

Echandía Castilla, Camilo, and Eduardo Bechara Gómez. 2006. "Conducta de la guerrilla durante el gobierno Uribe Vélez: De las lógicas de control territorial a las lógicas de control estratégico." *Análisis Político* 19 (57): 31–54.

Ecks, Stefan. 2005. "Pharmaceutical Citizenship: Antidepressant Marketing and the Promise of Demarginalization in India." *Anthropology & Medicine* 12 (3): 239–54. https://doi.org/10.1080/13648470500291360.

Ejército Nacional. 2013. "La Fuerza también tiene heroínas: El papel de la mujer en el Ejército colombiano." Ejército Nacional de Colombia. 2013. https://www.ejercito.mil.co/?idcategoria=349399.

———. 2016. "Así Se Forman Los Hombres de Las Fuerzas Especiales de Colombia. Conoce Aquí Los Pormenores Del Curso." 2016. http://www.fuerzasmilitares.org/notas/colombia/ejercito-nacional/7034-ffee-colombia.html.

———. 2018. "La Primera Mujer de Infantería En La Historia del Ejército Nacional." April. https://www.esmic.edu.co/sala_prensa/noticias/la_primera_mujer_infanteria_2681_2681.

———. n.d.-a. "Preguntas Frecuentes." Comando de Reclutamiento y Control Reservas. Accessed May 16, 2019. https://www.libretamilitar.mil.co/modules/Help/Faqs.

———. n.d.-b. "Preguntas frecuentes—Ejercito Nacional de Colombia." Ejército Nacional de Colombia. Accessed May 16, 2019. https://www.ejercito.mil.co/servicio_ciudadano/preguntas_frecuentes_334201.

Elbe, Stefan, Anne Roemer-Mahler, and Christopher Long. 2015. "Medical Countermeasures for National Security: A New Government Role in the Pharmaceuticalization of Society." *Social Science & Medicine (1982)* 131 (April): 263–71. https://doi.org/10.1016/j.socscimed.2014.04.035.

El Colombiano. 2005. "Brasil Investiga Venta de Medicinas a Las Farc." *El Colombiano*. http://www.elcolombiano.com/olac_medicinas_jj_25032005-KVEC_AO_4227085.

El Espectador. 2014. "Incautan Medicamentos de Las Farc En Huila." *El Espectador*, April 9, 2014. http://www.elespectador.com/noticias/judicial/incautan-medicamentos-de-farc-huila-articulo-485968.

———. 2018. "Homicidios en Colombia: la tasa más baja en los últimos 42 años se dio en 2017." *El Espectador*, January 21, 2018, sec. Judicial. https://www.elespectador.com/noticias/judicial/homicidios-en-colombia-la-tasa-mas-baja-en-los-ultimos-42-anos-se-dio-en-2017-articulo-734526.

———. 2019. "Denuncian presuntas 'batidas' del Ejército en Bogotá." *El Espectador*, August 5, 2019. https://www.elespectador.com/noticias/bogota/denuncian-presuntas-batidas-del-ejercito-en-bogota-articulo-874565.

———. 2021. "Policía y Ejército, entre las entidades con más casos de corrupción en el Gobierno." *El Espectador*, December 2, 2021. https://www.elespectador.com/judicial/policia-y

-ejercito-entre-las-entidades-con-mas-casos-de-corrupcion-en-el-gobierno-informe-de-corrupcion-en-colombia/.

El Nuevo Siglo. 2011. "Contrabando, tragamonedas y extorsión: trío diabólico." *El Nuevo Siglo*, September 16, 2011. http://www.elnuevosiglo.com.co/articulos/9-2011-contrabando-tragamonedas-y-extorsion-trio-diabolico.

El Tiempo. 2001. "Extorsiones a Nombre de la Guerrilla." *El Tiempo*, February 16, 2001. http://www.eltiempo.com/archivo/documento/MAM-620072.

———. 2004a. "Alerta por aumento de leishmaniasis." *El Tiempo*, August 21, 2004. https://www.eltiempo.com/archivo/documento/MAM-1568814.

———. 2004b. "Plan Patriota y la leishmaniasis." *El Tiempo*, November 2, 2004. https://www.eltiempo.com/archivo/documento/MAM-1506269.

———. 2004c. "Leishmaniasis golpea a las filas." *El Tiempo*, November 3, 2004. http://www.eltiempo.com/archivo/documento/MAM-1509107.

———. 2005a. "Leishmaniasis y minas dejan por fuera de combate a 4000 militares." *El Tiempo*, February 5, 2005. https://www.eltiempo.com/archivo/documento/MAM-1676376.

———. 2005b. "Leishmaniasis, enemigo mortal en la selva." *El Tiempo*, March 29, 2005. http://www.eltiempo.com/archivo/documento/MAM-1635174.

———. 2006a. "Insecticida contra leishmaniasis hasta en calzoncillos y calcetines militares." *El Tiempo*, January 25, 2006. https://www.eltiempo.com/archivo/documento/MAM-1895136.

———. 2006b. "Guerra En Nariño Es Por El Rambo de Las Farc." *El Tiempo*, July 25, 2006. http://www.eltiempo.com/archivo/documento/MAM-2113864.

———. 2007a. "La leishmaniasis es la principal enfermedad que afecta al Ejército, hace un mes murió un uniformado." *El Tiempo*, June 19, 2007. http://www.eltiempo.com/archivo/documento/CMS-3601632.

———. 2007b. "En Duitama (Boyacá) funciona centro de recuperación de leishmaniasis." *El Tiempo*, July 1, 2007. http://www.eltiempo.com/archivo/documento/CMS-3619806.

———. 2008a. "¿Milicianos Importados Tras Seguidilla de Petardos?" *El Tiempo*, June 14, 2008. http://www.eltiempo.com/archivo/documento/MAM-2974303.

———. 2008b. "La leishmaniasis: una enfermedad que causa estigma social." *El Tiempo*, July 9, 2008. http://www.eltiempo.com/archivo/documento/CMS-4369071.

———. 2009a. "Se Desmovilizan Ocho Integrantes Del Frente Aurelio Rodríguez de Las Farc." *El Tiempo*, January 29, 2009. http://www.eltiempo.com/archivo/documento/CMS-4782583.

———. 2009b. "Cavernas Naturales Donde Se Escondía El 'Mono Jojoy' Fueron Descubiertas Por La Fuerza Omega." *El Tiempo*, February 28, 2009. http://www.eltiempo.com/archivo/documento/CMS-4848582.

———. 2009c. "Ejército Rescató Ayer a Otro Secuestrado." *El Tiempo*, March 1, 2009. http://www.eltiempo.com/archivo/documento/MAM-3340454.

———. 2013. "Editorial: Contra las batidas." *El Tiempo*, December 12, 2013. https://www.eltiempo.com/archivo/documento/CMS-13282567.

Emanuelsson, Dick. 2012. La guerrillera Susana que sobrevivió el bombardeo del campamento de Raúl Reyes: "En esta lucha unos vamos, otros nos quedaremos en el camino y otros continuarán la lucha que llevamos" Anncol. http://2014.anncol.eu/index.php/opinion/dick-emanuelsson-anncol/1034-dec-12-video-la-guerrillera-susana-que-sobrevivio-el-bombardeo-del-campamento-de-raul-reyes-en-esta-lucha-unos-vamos-otros-nos-quedaremos-en-el-camino-y-otros-continuaran-la-lucha-que-llevamos.

"Engelver García Pallares." n.d. Vidas Silenciadas. Accessed May 26, 2019. https://vidassilenciadas.org/victimas/37346/.

Enloe, Cynthia. 2023. *Twelve Feminist Lessons of War*. Berkeley: University of California Press.

Espinosa, Mariola. 2009. *Epidemic Invasions: Yellow Fever and the Limits of Cuban Independence, 1878–1930*. Chicago: University of Chicago Press.

ESPRO. 2019. "Costos—ESPRO." ESPRO. Ejército Nacional de Colombia. May 11, 2019. https://www.espro.mil.co/escuela_soldados_profesionales/incorporaciones/costos.

———. n.d. "Reseña Histórica—ESPRO." Escuela de Soldados Profesionales. Accessed June 1, 2019. https://www.espro.mil.co/escuela_soldados_profesionales/quienes_somos/resena_historica.

Fassin, Didier. 2007. *When Bodies Remember: Experiences and Politics of AIDS in South Africa*. Berkeley: University of California Press.

———. 2008. "The Politics of Death: Race, War, Biopower and AIDS in the Post-Apartheid." In *Foucault on Politics, Security and War*, edited by Michael Dillon and Andrew W. Neal, 151–65. London: Palgrave Macmillan. https://doi.org/10.1057/9780230229846_8.

———. 2009. "A Violence of History: Accounting for AIDS in Post-Apartheid South Africa." In *Global Health in Times of Violence*, edited by Barbara Rylko-Bauer, Linda Whiteford, and Paul Farmer, 113–35. Santa Fe, NM: School for Advanced Research Press.

———. 2012. "That Obscure Object of Global Health." In *Medical Anthropology at the Intersections: Histories, Activisms, and Futures*, edited by Marcia C. Inhorn and Emily A. Wentzell, 95–115. Durham, NC: Duke University Press.

Fernandes Cota, Gláucia, Marcos Roberto de Sousa, Tatiani Oliveira Fereguetti, Priscila Said Saleme, Thais Kawagoe Alvarisa, and Ana Rabello. 2016. "The Cure Rate after Placebo or No Therapy in American Cutaneous Leishmaniasis: A Systematic Review and Meta-Analysis." *PLoS ONE* 11 (2): e0149697. https://doi.org/10.1371/journal.pone.0149697.

Fernández, Olga Lucía, Yira Diaz-Toro, Clemencia Ovalle, Liliana Valderrama, Sandra Muvdi, Isabel Rodríguez, María Adelaida Gomez, and Nancy Gore Saravia. 2014. "Miltefosine and Antimonial Drug Susceptibility of *Leishmania Viannia* Species and Populations in Regions of High Transmission in Colombia." *PLoS Neglected Tropical Diseases* 8 (5). https://doi.org/10.1371/journal.pntd.0002871.

Ferro, Cristina, Marla López, Patricia Fuya, Ligia Lugo, Juan Manuel Cordovez, and Camila González. 2015. "Spatial Distribution of Sand Fly Vectors and Eco-Epidemiology of Cutaneous Leishmaniasis Transmission in Colombia." *PLoS ONE* 10 (10). https://doi.org/10.1371/journal.pone.0139391.

Fidler, David P., and Lawrence O. Gostin. 2006. "The New International Health Regulations: An Historic Development for International Law and Public Health." *Journal of Law, Medicine & Ethics* 34 (1): 85–94.

Forero Angel, Ana María. 2017. "El Ejército Nacional de Colombia y sus heridas: Una aproximación a las narrativas militares de dolor y desilusión." *Antípoda*, September.

Fortun, Kim. 2009. "Scaling and Visualizing Multi-Sited Ethnography." In *Multi-Sited Ethnography: Theory, Praxis and Locality in Contemporary Research*, edited by Mark-Anthony Falzon, 73–85. Farnham: Ashgate.

Franco, Saúl. 2003. "Para que la salud sea pública: Algunas lecciones de la reforma de salud y seguridad social en Colombia." *Revista Gerencia y Políticas de Salud* 2 (4). http://www.redalyc.org/resumen.oa?id=54520406.

Franco, Saúl, Clara Mercedes Suarez, Claudia Beatriz Naranjo, Liliana Carolina Báez, and Patricia Rozo. 2006. "The Effects of the Armed Conflict on the Life and Health in Colombia." *Ciência & Saúde Coletiva* 11 (2): 349–61.

French, Martin, and Eric Mykhalovskiy. 2013. "Public Health Intelligence and the Detection of Potential Pandemics." *Sociology of Health & Illness* 35 (2): 174–87. https://doi.org/10.1111/j.1467-9566.2012.01536.x.

Fundación Ideas para la Paz. 2013. "Dinámicas del Conflicto Armado en Tolima y su Impacto Humanitario." http://archive.ideaspaz.org/images/DocumentoMonitoreo_ConflictoArmado_Tolima_Julio2013.pdf.

Fundación Ideas para la Paz and Oficina del Alto Comisionado para la Paz. 2019. "La Reincorporación de Los Excombatientes de Las FARC." http://ideaspaz.org/especiales/infografias/excombatientes.html?fbclid=IwAR0GwfxvU0gQEhCMP1Zbi-7BF5N8t4hDl_YoY86dldVuNYlaUOVUc6vaJdc.

Gabe, Jonathan, Simon Williams, Paul Martin, and Catherine Coveney. 2015. "Pharmaceuticals and Society: Power, Promises and Prospects." *Social Science & Medicine* 131 (April): 193–98. https://doi.org/10.1016/j.socscimed.2015.02.031.

Gallón, Gustavo. 2005. "Los Riesgos de Una Desenfocada Política Antiterrorista En Colombia." In *La Reforma Política Del Estado En Colombia: Una Salida Integral a La Crisis*, by Miguel Cárdenas, 121–53. Bogotá: Cerec-Fescol.

Gallup Colombia. 2017. "Gallup Poll #117 Colombia Febrero 2017." https://www.eltiempo.com/contenido/politica/gobierno/ARCHIVO/ARCHIVO-16832164-0.pdf.

García, María Isabel. 1994. "La guerrina colombiana, al asalto de la ciudad." *El País*, September 16, 1994, sec. Internacional. https://elpais.com/diario/1994/09/16/internacional/779666418_850215.html.

Geest, Sjaak van der. 2006. "Anthropology and the Pharmaceutical Nexus." *Anthropological Quarterly* 79 (2): 303–14.

Geissler, P. W. 2013. "Public Secrets in Public Health: Knowing Not to Know While Making Scientific Knowledge." *American Ethnologist* 40 (1): 13–34. https://doi.org/10.1111/amet.12002.

Geltzer, Anna. 2009. "When the Standards Aren't Standard: Evidence-Based Medicine in the Russian Context." *Social Science & Medicine* 68 (3): 526–32. https://doi.org/10.1016/j.socscimed.2008.10.029.

Ghert-Zand, Renee. 2024. "Sandfly-Borne Parasitic Disease Has Affected at Least 100 IDF Troops in Gaza," January 2, 2024. https://www.timesofisrael.com/sandfly-borne-parasitic-disease-has-affected-at-least-100-idf-troops-in-gaza/.

Ghobarah, Hazem Adam, Paul Huth, and Bruce Russett. 2004. "The Post-War Public Health Effects of Civil Conflict." *Social Science & Medicine* 59 (4): 869–84. https://doi.org/10.1016/j.socscimed.2003.11.043.

Gibson, Mary E. 1983. "The Identification of Kala-Azar and the Discovery of Leishmania Donovani." *Medical History* 27 (2): 203–13.

Giraud, Eva Haifa. 2019. *What Comes after Entanglement?: Activism, Anthropocentrism, and an Ethics of Exclusion*. Durham, NC: Duke University Press.

Goffman, Erving. 1986. *Stigma: Notes on the Management of Spoiled Identity*. New York: Touchstone.

Gómez-Restrepo, Carlos, Nathalie Tamayo-Martínez, Giancarlo Buitrago, Carol Cristina Guarnizo-Herreño, Nathaly Garzón-Orjuela, Javier Eslava-Schmalbach, Esther de Vries, Herney Rengifo, Andrea Rodríguez, and Carlos Javier Rincón. 2016. "Violencia Por

Conflicto Armado y Prevalencias de Trastornos Del Afecto, Ansiedad y Problemas Mentales En La Población Adulta Colombiana." *Revista Colombiana de Psiquiatría* 45 (December): 147–53. https://doi.org/10.1016/j.rcp.2016.11.001.

González, Aida M., María Teresa Solis-Soto, and Katja Radon. 2017. "Leishmaniasis: Who Uses Personal Protection among Military Personnel in Colombia?" *Annals of Global Health* 83:519–23.

González, Fernán E. 2003. "Hacia Una Mirada Más Compleja de La Violencia Colombiana." In *Violencia Política En Colombia: De La Nación Fragmentada a La Construcción Del Estado*, edited by Fernán E. González, Ingrid Bolívar, and Teófilo Vázquez, 17–46. Bogotá: CINEP.

González, María Fernanda. 2017. "La «posverdad» en el plebiscito por la paz en Colombia." *Nueva Sociedad*, no. 269, 114–26.

Goodwin, L. G. 1995. "Pentostam (Sodium Stibogluconate); A 50-Year Personal Reminiscence." *Transactions of the Royal Society of Tropical Medicine and Hygiene* 89:339–41.

Gray, Harriet. 2015. "The Trauma Risk Management Approach to Post-Traumatic Stress Disorder in the British Military: Masculinity, Biopolitics and Depoliticisation." *Feminist Review* 111 (1): 109–23. https://doi.org/10.1057/fr.2015.23.

Green, Linda. 1994. "Fear as a Way of Life." *Cultural Anthropology*, 227–56.

Greene, Jeremy A. 2011. "Making Medicines Essential: The Emergent Centrality of Pharmaceuticals in Global Health." *BioSocieties* 6 (1): 10–33. https://doi.org/10.1057/biosoc.2010.39.

Greene, Jeremy A., and Sergio Sismondo. 2015. "Introduction." In *The Pharmaceutical Studies Reader*, edited by Sergio Sismondo and Jeremy A. Greene, 1–16. Chichester: Wiley-Blackwell.

Greenwood, David. 2008. *Antimicrobial Drugs: Chronicle of a Twentieth Century Medical Triumph*. Oxford: Oxford University Press.

Guarnizo Alvarez, José. 2010. "Glucantime, La Otra Disputa de La Guerra." *El Colombiano*, August 15, 2010. http://www.elcolombiano.com/glucantime_la_otra_disputa_de_la_guerra-CEEC_100741.

Haldar, Arun Kumar, Pradip Sen, and Syamal Roy. 2011. "Use of Antimony in the Treatment of Leishmaniasis: Current Status and Future Directions." *Molecular Biology International* 2011:1–23. https://doi.org/10.4061/2011/571242.

Haraoui, Louis-Patrick. 2007. "The Orientalist Sore: Biomedical Discourses, Capital and Urban Warfare in the Colonial Present." Montréal: Université de Montréal. https://papyrus.bib.umontreal.ca/xmlui/handle/1866/7343.

Haraway, Donna. 2003. *The Companion Species Manifesto: Dogs, People, and Significant Otherness*. Chicago: Prickly Paradigm Press.

Harrison, M. 1996. "The Medicalization of War—The Militarization of Medicine." *Social History of Medicine* 9 (2): 267–76.

Harrison, Mark, and Sung Vin Yim. 2017. "War on Two Fronts: The Fight against Parasites in Korea and Vietnam." *Medical History* 61 (3): 401–23. https://doi.org/10.1017/mdh.2017.35.

Hayden, Cori. 2007. "A Generic Solution?: Pharmaceuticals and the Politics of the Similar in Mexico." *Current Anthropology* 48 (4): 475–95. https://doi.org/10.1086/518301.

He, Mengchang, Xiangqin Wang, Fengchang Wu, and Zhiyou Fu. 2012. "Antimony Pollution in China." *Science of the Total Environment*, Special Section: Reviews of Trace Metal Pollution in China, 421–422 (April): 41–50. https://doi.org/10.1016/j.scitotenv.2011.06.009.

Henao, Juan Carlos, and Carolina Isaza. 2018. *Corrupción en Colombia Tomo I: Corrupción, Política y Sociedad*. Bogotá: Universidad Externado de Colombia.

Henry, Doug. 2006. "Violence and the Body: Somatic Expressions of Trauma and Vulnerability during War." *Medical Anthropology Quarterly* 20 (3): 379–98.

Herrera, Giovanny, Aníbal Teherán, Iván Pradilla, Mauricio Vera, and Juan David Ramírez. 2018. "Geospatial-Temporal Distribution of Tegumentary Leishmaniasis in Colombia (2007–2016)." *PLoS Neglected Tropical Diseases* 12 (4). https://doi.org/10.1371/journal.pntd.0006419.

Herrera Durán, Natalia. 2015. "Un filósofo sin libreta militar." *El Espectador*. February 28, 2015. https://www.elespectador.com/noticias/bogota/un-filosofo-sin-libreta-militar-articulo-546744.

Hochman, Gilberto, María Silvia Di Liscia, and Steven Palmer. 2012. *Patologías de la patria: Enfermedades, enfermos y nación en América Latina*. Buenos Aires: Lugar Editorial.

Howell, Alison. 2011. *Madness in International Relations: Psychology, Security, and the Global Governance of Mental Health*. New York: Routledge.

Ibañez Sarco, Monica. 2015. "Colombia: Lo que en su momento fue símbolo de guerra hoy sirve de lienzo para la paz." *Aleteia* (blog). February 1, 2015. http://es.aleteia.org/2015/02/01/colombia-lo-que-en-su-momento-fue-simbolo-de-guerra-hoy-sirve-de-lienzo-para-la-paz/.

Idler, Annette. 2019. *Borderland Battles: Violence, Crime, and Governance at the Edges of Colombia's War*. Oxford: Oxford University Press.

IISS. 2005. "Chapter Seven: Caribbean and Latin America." *Military Balance* 105 (1): 315–58. https://doi.org/10.1080/04597220500387670.

———. 2019. "Chapter Eight: Latin America and the Caribbean." *Military Balance* 119 (1): 380–437. https://doi.org/10.1080/04597222.2018.1561034.

Inci, Rahime, Perihan Ozturk, Mehmet Kamil Mulayim, Kemal Ozyurt, Emine Tugba Alatas, and Mehmet Fatih Inci. 2015. "Effect of the Syrian Civil War on Prevalence of Cutaneous Leishmaniasis in Southeastern Anatolia, Turkey." *Medical Science Monitor* 21:2100–2104. https://doi.org/10.12659/MSM.893977.

INS. 2017. "Protocolo de Vigilancia En Salud Pública, Leishmaniasis." https://www.ins.gov.co/buscador-eventos/ZIKA%20Lineamientos/PRO%20Leishmaniasis.pdf.

———. 2019. "Lineamientos Nacionales 2019—Vigilancia y Control En Salud Pública." https://www.ins.gov.co/Direcciones/Vigilancia/Lineamientosydocumentos/Lineamientos%202019.pdf.

INS and ONS. 2017. "Consecuencias Del Conflicto Armado En La Salud de Colombia." Technical report 9. Bogotá. https://www.ins.gov.co/Direcciones/ONS/Informes/9%20Consecuencias%20del%20Conflicto%20Armado%20en%20la%20Salud%20en%20Colombia.pdf.

Iza Rodríguez, José Alejandro, Shirley Natali Iza Rodríguez, and Mario Javier Olivera. 2021. "Leishmaniasis in the Colombian Post-Conflict Era: A Descriptive Study from 2004 to 2019." *Revista Da Sociedade Brasileira de Medicina Tropical* 54: e0612-2020. https://doi.org/10.1590/0037-8682-0612-2020.

Jackson, Michael. 2002. *The Politics of Storytelling: Violence, Transgression and Intersubjectivity*. Copenhagen Denmark: Museum Tusculanum.

Jacobson, Raymond L. 2011. "Leishmaniasis in an Era of Conflict in the Middle East." *Vector-Borne and Zoonotic Diseases* 11 (3): 247–58. https://doi.org/10.1089/vbz.2010.0068.

Jaramillo, Hernán, Carolina Lopera, Beatriz González, and Andrés Vecino. 2009. "Impacto Del Financiamiento En Investigación En Salud, Colciencias 1970–2007." Bogotá: Colciencias.

Jimeno, Myriam. 2001. "Violence and Social Life in Colombia." *Critique of Anthropology* 21 (3): 221–46. https://doi.org/10.1177/0308275X0102100302.

Jogas Junior, Denis Guedes, and Jaime Larry Benchimol. 2020. "Leishmaniose Tegumentar Americana: Gênese e Consolidação de Um Conceito." In *Uma História Das Leishmanioses No Novo Mundo: Fins Do Século XIX Aos Anos 1960*, edited by Jaime Larry Benchimol and Denis Guedes Jogas Junior, 29–91. Rio de Janeiro: Fiocruz.

Kamhawi, Shaden. 2017. "The Yin and Yang of Leishmaniasis Control." *PLoS Neglected Tropical Diseases* 11 (4): e0005529.

Kellman, Shannon. 2022. "War-Torn Ukraine Is Also an HIV and Tuberculosis Hot Spot." *Foreign Policy*, August 31, 2022. https://foreignpolicy.com/2022/08/31/ukraine-russia-war-hiv-tuberculosis-epidemic-medication-health-care/.

King, Nicholas. 2002. "Security, Disease, Commerce: Ideologies of Postcolonial Global Health." *Social Studies of Science* 32:763–89.

———. 2004. "The Scale Politics of Emerging Diseases." *Osiris* 19:62–76.

Kitchen, Lynn W., Kendra L. Lawrence, and Russell E. Coleman. 2009. "The Role of the United States Military in the Development of Vector Control Products, Including Insect Repellents, Insecticides, and Bed Nets." *Journal of Vector Ecology* 34 (1): 50–61.

Kluger, Jeffrey, and Tara Law. 2022. "Polio Makes a Comeback in Ukraine as War Halts Vaccinations." *Time*, March 9, 2022. https://time.com/6155963/polio-ukraine-war/.

Knaapen, Loes. 2014. "Evidence-Based Medicine or Cookbook Medicine? Addressing Concerns over the Standardization of Care." *Sociology Compass* 8 (6): 823–36. https://doi.org/10.1111/soc4.12184.

Koopman, Sara. 2017. "Peace." In *International Encyclopedia of Geography: People, the Earth, Environment and Technology*, edited by Douglas Richardson, Noel Castree, Michael F. Goodchild, Audrey Kobayashi, Weidong Liu, and Richard A. Marston, 1–4. Oxford: John Wiley & Sons. https://doi.org/10.1002/9781118786352.wbieg1175.

Kosek, Jake. 2010. "Ecologies of Empire: On the New Uses of the Honeybee." *Cultural Anthropology* 25 (4): 650–78. https://doi.org/10.1111/j.1548-1360.2010.01073.x.

Kreutzer, R. D., A. Corredor, G. Grimaldi, M. Grogl, E. D. Rowton, D. G. Young, A. Morales, D. McMahon-Pratt, H. Guzman, and R. B. Tesh. 1991. "Characterization of Leishmania Colombiensis Sp. n (Kinetoplastida: Trypanosomatidae), a New Parasite Infecting Humans, Animals, and Phlebotomine Sand Flies in Colombia and Panama." *American Journal of Tropical Medicine and Hygiene* 44 (6): 662–75. https://doi.org/10.4269/ajtmh.1991.44.662.

Kroc Institute. 2023. "Implementation of the Colombian Peace Accord Reaches Its Sixth Year." https://curate.nd.edu/articles/report/Implementation_of_the_Colombian_Peace_Accord_Reaches_its_Sixth_Year/24870264?file=43760970.

Lachenal, Guillaume. 2017. *The Lomidine Files: The Untold Story of a Medical Disaster in Colonial Africa*. Baltimore: Johns Hopkins University Press.

Lakoff, Andrew. 2010. "Two Regimes of Global Health." *Humanity: An International Journal of Human Rights, Humanitarianism, and Development* 1 (1): 59–79. https://doi.org/10.1353/hum.2010.0001.

———. 2017. *Unprepared: Global Health in a Time of Emergency*. Oakland: University of California Press.

La Nación. 2005. "Crisis en sur de Colombia por enfrentamientos armados." *La Nación*. July 31, 2005. https://www.nacion.com/el-mundo/crisis-en-sur-de-colombia-por-enfrentamientos-armados/7FP3KHPIKRDEBIKC3L5TGN6G4Q/story/.

Landecker, Hannah. 2016. "Antibiotic Resistance and the Biology of History." *Body & Society* 22 (4): 19–52. https://doi.org/10.1177/1357034X14561341.

Langston, Nancy. 2010. *Toxic Bodies: Hormone Disruptors and the Legacy of DES*. New Haven, CT: Yale University Press.

La Patria. 2013. "Denuncie Sin Temor Las Extorsiones, La Mayoría Son Desde Las Cárceles." *La Patria*, December 14, 2013. http://www.lapatria.com/sucesos/denuncie-sin-temor-las-extorsiones-la-mayoria-son-desde-las-carceles-50779.

Latour, Bruno. 1992. "Where Are the Missing Masses? The Sociology of a Few Mundane Artifacts." In *Shaping Technology / Building Society*, edited by Wiebe E. Bijker and John Law, 225–58. Cambridge, MA: MIT Press.

———. 1993. *We Have Never Been Modern*. Cambridge, MA: Harvard University Press.

Law, John. 2008. "Actor Network Theory and Material Semiotics." In *The New Blackwell Companion to Social Theory*, edited by Bryan S. Turner, 141–58. John Wiley & Sons. https://doi.org/10.1002/9781444304992.ch7.

Layne, Linda L. 2000. "The Cultural Fix: An Anthropological Contribution to Science and Technology Studies." *Science, Technology, & Human Values* 25 (3): 352–79. https://doi.org/10.1177/016224390002500305.

Leal Buitrago, Francisco. 2006. "Las deudas de la seguridad." *El Tiempo*, July 24, 2006. https://www.eltiempo.com/archivo/documento/MAM-2112116.

———. 2011. "Una Visión de la Seguridad Democrática en Colombia." *Análisis Político* 24 (73): 3–36.

LeGrand, Catherine C., Luis van Isschot, and Pilar Riaño-Alcalá. 2017. "Land, Justice, and Memory: Challenges for Peace in Colombia." *Canadian Journal of Latin American and Caribbean Studies / Revue Canadienne Des Études Latino-Américaines et Caraïbes* 42 (3): 259–76. https://doi.org/10.1080/08263663.2017.1378381.

Lesho, Emil P., Glenn W. Wortmann, Ronald C. Neafie, and Naomi E. Aronson. 2004. "Cutaneous Leishmaniasis: Battling the Baghdad Boil." *Federal Practitioner*, 59–67.

Levy, Barry S., and Victor W. Sidel, eds. 2007. *War and Public Health*. New York: Oxford University Press.

Lezaun, J., and C. M. Montgomery. 2015. "The Pharmaceutical Commons: Sharing and Exclusion in Global Health Drug Development." *Science, Technology & Human Values* 40 (1): 3–29. https://doi.org/10.1177/0162243914542349.

Liboiron, Max, Manuel Tironi, and Nerea Calvillo. 2018. "Toxic Politics: Acting in a Permanently Polluted World." *Social Studies of Science* 48 (3): 331–49. https://doi.org/10.1177/0306312718783087.

Linker, Beth. 2011. *War's Waste: Rehabilitation in World War I America*. Chicago: University of Chicago Press.

Llanera. 2011. "En Villavicencio Incautan Medicamentos Destinados a La Guerrilla. Estaban Destinados a Combatir La Leishmaniasis—Llanera.Com—Un Solo Llano." *Llanera*, March 25, 2011. http://llanera.com/?id=12007.

Lock, Margaret. 1995. *Encounters with Aging: Mythologies of Menopause in Japan and North America*. Berkeley: University of California Press.

Lock, Margaret, and Vinh-Kim Nguyen. 2010. *An Anthropology of Biomedicine*. Chichester, UK: Wiley-Blackwell.

Lockwood, Jeffrey. 2010. *Six-Legged Soldiers: Using Insects as Weapons of War*. Oxford: Oxford University Press.

López, Liliana, Claudia Cruz, Gonzalo Godoy, Sara M. Robledo, and Iván D. Vélez. 2013. "Thermoterapy Effective and Safer than Miltefosine in the Treatment of Cutaneous Leishmaniasis in Colombia." *Revista Do Instituto de Medicina Tropical de São Paulo* 55 (3): 197–204. https://doi.org/10.1590/S0036-46652013000300011.

López, Liliana, Martha Robayo, Margarita Vargas, and Iván D. Vélez. 2012. "Thermotherapy. An Alternative for the Treatment of American Cutaneous Leishmaniasis." *Trials* 13 (1): 58. https://doi.org/10.1186/1745-6215-13-58.

López, Liliana, Iván Vélez, Claudia Asela, Claudia Cruz, Fabiana Alves, Sara Robledo, and Byron Arana. 2018. "A Phase II Study to Evaluate the Safety and Efficacy of Topical 3% Amphotericin B Cream (Anfoleish) for the Treatment of Uncomplicated Cutaneous Leishmaniasis in Colombia." *PLOS Neglected Tropical Diseases* 12 (7): e0006653. https://doi.org/10.1371/journal.pntd.0006653.

Lyons, Kristina M. 2020. *Vital Decomposition: Soil Practitioners and Life Politics*. Durham, NC: Duke University Press.

Lyons, Kristina M., Lina Pinto-García, and Daniel Ruiz Serna. 2019. "Hacia una comprensión del conflicto y la paz en Colombia más allá de lo humano." *Maguaré* 33 (2): 15–22. https://doi.org/10.15446/mag.v33n2.88069.

MacLeish, Kenneth. 2013. *Making War at Fort Hood: Life and Uncertainty in a Military Community*. Princeton, NJ: Princeton University Press.

———. 2015. "The Ethnography of Good Machines." *Critical Military Studies* 1 (1): 11–22. https://doi.org/10.1080/23337486.2014.973680.

Majeed, B., J. Sobel, A. Nawar, S. Badri, and H. Muslim. 2013. "The Persisting Burden of Visceral Leishmaniasis in Iraq: Data of the National Surveillance System, 1990–2009." *Epidemiology and Infection* 141 (2): 443–46. https://doi.org/10.1017/S0950268812000556.

Marcus, George E. 1995. "Ethnography in/of the World System: The Emergence of Multi-Sited Ethnography." *Annual Review of Anthropology*, 95–117.

Martínez-Valencia, Alvaro J., Carlos Frisherald Daza-Rivera, Mariana Rosales-Chilama, Alexandra Cossio, Elkin J. Casadiego Rincón, Mayur M. Desai, Nancy Gore Saravia, and María Adelaida Gómez. 2017. "Clinical and Parasitological Factors in Parasite Persistence after Treatment and Clinical Cure of Cutaneous Leishmaniasis." *PLoS Neglected Tropical Diseases* 11 (7). https://doi.org/10.1371/journal.pntd.0005713.

Masco, Joseph. 2006. *The Nuclear Borderlands: The Manhattan Project in Post-Cold War New Mexico*. Princeton, NJ: Princeton University Press.

———. 2014. *The Theater of Operations: National Security Affect from the Cold War to the War on Terror*. Durham, NC: Duke University Press.

Masse, Frederic. 2011. "¿Bandas Criminales o Neoparamilitares?" *Foreign Affairs* 11 (2): 42–49.

McCallum, R. I. 1999. *Antimony in Medical History: An Account of the Medical Uses of Antimony and Its Compounds Since Early Times to the Present*. Edinburgh: Pentland.

McGoey, Linsey. 2015. *No Such Thing as a Free Gift: The Gates Foundation and the Price of Philanthropy*. Brooklyn, NY: Verso.

McReynolds-Perez, Julia A. 2014. "Misoprostol for the Masses: The Activist-Led Proliferation of Pharmaceutical Abortion in Argentina." PhD diss., University of Wisconsin–Madison. http://proquest.com/docview/1835182231/abstract.

Medina, Harvey Yecid. 2007a. "Por Leishmaniasis Han Sido Atendidos Cerca de 3.000 Hombres En Batallón Silva Plazas, de Duitama." *El Tiempo*, June 19, 2007. http://www.eltiempo.com/archivo/documento/CMS-3601631.

———. 2007b. "En Duitama (Boyacá) Funciona Centro de Recuperación de Leishmaniasis." *El Tiempo*, July 1, 2007. http://www.eltiempo.com/archivo/documento/CMS-3619806.

Ministerio de Defensa, Ministerio de Salud, Instituto Nacional de Salud, and INVIMA. 2017. "Lineamientos generales para el fortalecimiento de la prevención, vigilancia y control de eventos de interés en salud pública en comandos – unidades militares y policiales." https://www.minsalud.gov.co/sites/rid/Lists/BibliotecaDigital/RIDE/VS/PP/PAI/Lineamientos-eventos-interes-salud-publica-comandos-mlitares-policiales.pdf.

MinSalud. 1998. "Acuerdo No. 117 de 1998." https://www.minsalud.gov.co/Normatividad_Nuevo/ACUERDO%20117%20DE%201998.pdf.

———. 2010. "Guía Para La Atención Clínica Integral Del Paciente Con Leishmaniasis." http://www.ins.gov.co/temas-de-interes/Leishmaniasis%20viceral/02%20Clinica%20Leishmaniasis.pdf.

———. 2018. "Lineamientos Para La Atención Clínica Integral de Leishmaniasis En Colombia." https://www.minsalud.gov.co/sites/rid/Lists/BibliotecaDigital/RIDE/VS/PP/PAI/Lineamientos-leishmaniasis.pdf.

———. 2022. "Plan Nacional de Salud Rural." https://portalparalapaz.gov.co/wp-content/uploads/2022/07/Archivo-Digital-08-Plan-Nacional-de-Salud.pdf.

———. 2023. "Lineamientos de Atención Clínica Integral Para Leishmaniasis En Colombia." https://www.minsalud.gov.co/sites/rid/Lists/BibliotecaDigital/RIDE/VS/PP/PAI/Lineamientos-leishmaniasis.pdf.

MinSalud and INS. 2017. "Protocolo de Vigilancia En Salud Pública—Leishmaniasis, Código 420, 430 y 440." http://www.dadiscartagena.gov.co/images/docs/saludpublica/vigilancia/protocolos/p2018/pro_leishmaniasis_2018.pdf.

Minuto 30. 2013. "La leishmaniasis, una enfermedad 'que camina' con el conflicto armado en Antioquia." *Minuto 30*, August 16, 2013. https://www.minuto30.com/la-leishmaniasis-una-enfermedad-que-camina-con-el-conflicto-armado-en-antioquia/174556/.

MOE and Fundación Ciudad Abierta. 2017. "Tercer Informe Aprendizaje Desde Los Territorios." https://moe.org.co/wp-content/uploads/2017/06/Descargue-el-informe-completo-de-observaci%C3%B3n-a-las-Zonas-Veredales-Transitorias-de-Normalizaci%C3%B3n-2017-2.pdf.

Molano Bravo, Alfredo. 2001. *Desterrados: Crónicas del desarraigo*. Bogotá: El Áncora Editores.

———. 2005a. *Aguas Arriba: Entre la Coca y el Oro*. Bogotá: El Áncora Editores.

———. 2005b. "Perversa Estrategia." *Agencia Prensa Rural*, April 9, 2005. http://www.prensarural.org/molano20050409.htm.

Monsalve Gaviria, Ricardo. 2017. "Ubicada otra caleta con armamento y medicamentos del Clan del Golfo." *El Colombiano*, April 27, 2017. https://www.elcolombiano.com/colombia/paz-y-derechos-humanos/ejercito-incauta-armamento-del-clan-del-golfo-IY6405138.

Montoya-Lerma, James, Yezid A. Solarte, Gloria Isabel Giraldo-Calderón, Martha L. Quiñones, Freddy Ruiz-López, Richard C. Wilkerson, and Ranulfo González. 2011. "Malaria Vector Species in Colombia—A Review." *Memorias Do Instituto Oswaldo Cruz* 106 (Suppl. 1): 223–38.

Moore, Kelly. 2013. *Disrupting Science: Social Movements, American Scientists, and the Politics of the Military, 1945–1975*. Princeton, NJ: Princeton University Press.

Mora-Gámez, Fredy. 2023. "The Official Record of Victims as a Bordering Technology: Knowledge and (in)Visibilities in Post-Conflict Colombia." *Science as Culture* 32 (3): 344–62. https://doi.org/10.1080/09505431.2023.2221278.

Moreno, Mónica Cecilia Moreno, and María Victoria López López. 2009. "La Salud Como Derecho En Colombia. 1999–2007." *Revista Gerencia y Políticas de Salud* 8 (16): 133–52.

Murguía, Adriana, Teresa Ordorika, and León F. Lendo. 2016. "El Estudio de Los Procesos de Medicalización En América Latina." *História, Ciências, Saúde-Manguinhos* 23 (3): 635–51. https://doi.org/10.1590/S0104-59702016005000009.

Mykhalovskiy, Eric, and Lorna Weir. 2004. "The Problem of Evidence-Based Medicine: Directions for Social Science." *Social Science & Medicine (1982)* 59 (5): 1059–69. https://doi.org/10.1016/j.socscimed.2003.12.002.

Nading, Alex M. 2014. *Mosquito Trails: Ecology, Health, and the Politics of Entanglement*. Oakland: University of California Press.

———. 2017. "Local Biologies, Leaky Things, and the Chemical Infrastructure of Global Health." *Medical Anthropology* 36 (2): 141–56. https://doi.org/10.1080/01459740.2016.1186672.

———. 2020. "Living in a Toxic World." *Annual Review of Anthropology* 49 (1): 209–24. https://doi.org/10.1146/annurev-anthro-010220-074557.

Narvaez, Leonidas. 2017. "Vías terciarias: Motor del desarrollo económico rural." *Revista de Ingeniería*, no. 45. http://www.redalyc.org/resumen.oa?id=121052004013.

Neill, Deborah. 2012. *Networks in Tropical Medicine: Internationalism, Colonialism, and the Rise of a Medical Specialty, 1890–1930*. Stanford, CA: Stanford University Press.

Newlands, Emma. 2013. " 'They Even Gave Us Oranges on One Occasion': Human Experimentation in the British Army during the Second World War." *War & Society* 32 (1): 19–63.

Nguyen, Vinh-Kim. 2010. *The Republic of Therapy: Triage and Sovereignty in West Africa's Time of AIDS*. Durham, NC: Duke University Press.

Nguyen, Vinh-Kim, Cyriaque Yapo Ako, Pascal Niamba, Aliou Sylla, and Issoufou Tiendrébéogo. 2007. "Adherence as Therapeutic Citizenship: Impact of the History of Access to Antiretroviral Drugs on Adherence to Treatment." *AIDS* 21 (October): S31. https://doi.org/10.1097/01.aids.0000298100.48990.58.

Nordstrom, Carolyn. 2004. *Shadows of War: Violence, Power, and International Profiteering in the Twenty-First Century*. Berkeley: University of California Press.

———. 2009. "Fault Lines." In *Global Health in Times of Violence*, edited by Barbara Rylko-Bauer, Linda Whiteford, and Paul Farmer, 63–87. School for Advanced Research Press.

Nunes, João. 2016. "Ebola and the Production of Neglect in Global Health." *Third World Quarterly* 37 (3): 542–56. https://doi.org/10.1080/01436597.2015.1124724.

Obregón, Diana. 1996. "The Social Construction of Leprosy in Colombia, 1884–1939." *Science, Technology and Society* 1 (1): 1–23. https://doi.org/10.1177/097172189600100102.

———. 2002. "Building National Medicine: Leprosy and Power in Colombia, 1870–1910." *Social History of Medicine* 15 (1): 89–108. https://doi.org/10.1093/shm/15.1.89.

Observatorio de Memoria y Conflicto. 2023. "Observatorio de Memoria y Conflicto—Contando la Guerra en Colombia." http://centrodememoriahistorica.gov.co/observatorio/.

Ocampo, C. B., M. C. Ferro, H. Cadena, R. Gongora, M. Pérez, C. H. Valderrama-Ardila, R. J. Quinnell, and N. Alexander. 2012. "Environmental Factors Associated with American Cutaneous Leishmaniasis in a New Andean Focus in Colombia." *Tropical Medicine & International Health: TM & IH* 17 (10): 1309–17. https://doi.org/10.1111/j.1365-3156.2012.03065.x.

Ogao, Emma. 2023. "'Disease Catastrophe' Looms in Sudan as Health Conditions Deteriorate, Medics Warn." *ABC News*, August 11, 2023. https://abcnews.go.com/International/disease-catastrophe-looms-sudan-health-conditions-deteriorate-medics/story?id=102125078.

Ojeda, Diana, and Lina Pinto-García. 2020. "La Militarización de La Vida Durante La Guerra, El 'Posconflicto' y La Pandemia de COVID-19." *Platypus, the CASTAC Blog* (blog). September 4, 2020. http://blog.castac.org/multilingual/la-militarizacion-de-la-vida-durante-la-guerra-el-posconflicto-y-la-pandemia-de-covid-19/.

O'Manique, Colleen. 2005. "The 'Securitisation' of HIV/AIDS in Sub-Saharan Africa: A Critical Feminist Lens." *Policy and Society* 24 (1): 24–47. https://doi.org/10.1016/S1449-4035(05)70048-5.

Oransky, Ivan. 2019. "Time to Say Goodbye to 'Statistically Significant' and Embrace Uncertainty, Say Statisticians." *Retraction Watch* (blog). March 21, 2019. https://retractionwatch.com/2019/03/21/time-to-say-goodbye-to-statistically-significant-and-embrace-uncertainty-say-statisticians/.

Ordóñez Matamoros, Gonzalo, Juan Pablo Centeno, Elisa Arond, Astrid Jaime, and Kennicher Arias. 2018. "Los Retos de La Política de Ciencia, Tecnología e Innovación En Colombia." In *Seguimiento y Análisis de Políticas Públicas En Colombia*, edited by Carlos Soto, 137–68. Bogotá: Universidad Externado de Colombia.

Organización Panamericana de la Salud. 2013. "Leishmaniasis En Las Américas: Recomendaciones Para El Tratamiento."

Orjuela Benavides, Julián Alfonso. 2017. "La Salud Pública En El Tránsito de La Guerra a La Construcción de Paz En El Municipio de La Macarena." Bogotá: Pontificia Universidad Javeriana.

Ospina, María. 2014. "Las Naturalezas de La Guerra: Topografías Violentas de Selva En La Narrativa Contemporánea Colombiana." *Revista de Crítica Literaria Latinoamericana* 40 (79): 243–64.

Ostrach, Bayla, and Merrill Singer. 2012. "Syndemics of War: Malnutrition-Infectious Disease Interactions and the Unintended Health Consequences of Intentional War Policies." *Annals of Anthropological Practice* 36 (2): 257–73. https://doi.org/10.1111/napa.12003.

Ovalle-Bracho, Clemencia, Diana Londoño-Barbosa, Jussep Salgado-Almario, and Camila González. 2019. "Evaluating the Spatial Distribution of Leishmania Parasites in Colombia from Clinical Samples and Human Isolates (1999 to 2016)." *PLOS ONE* 14 (3): e0214124. https://doi.org/10.1371/journal.pone.0214124.

Packard, Randall M. 2011. *The Making of a Tropical Disease: A Short History of Malaria*. Baltimore: Johns Hopkins University Press.

———. 2016. *A History of Global Health: Interventions into the Lives of Other Peoples*. Baltimore: Johns Hopkins University Press.

Padilla, Julio César, Fredy Eberto Lizarazo, Olga Lucía Murillo, Fernando Antonio Mendigaña, Edwin Pachón, and Mauricio Javier Vera. 2017. "Epidemiología de Las Principales Enfermedades Transmitidas Por Vectores En Colombia, 1990–2016." *Biomédica* 37 (2): 27–40.

PAHO. 2016. "Recommendations of the Expert Committee for the Selection and Inclusion of Medicines in the Pan American Health Organization's Strategic Fund 2015." http://iris.paho.org/xmlui/bitstream/handle/123456789/28205/9789275118849_eng.pdf?sequence=1&isAllowed=y.

———. 2018. "PAHO Strategic Fund." Pan American Health Organization/World Health Organization. https://www.paho.org/hq/index.php?option=com_content&view=article&id=12163:paho-strategic-fund&Itemid=42005&lang=en.

———. 2023a. "PAHO Strategic Fund." https://www.paho.org/en/paho-strategic-fund.

———. 2023b. "PAHO Strategic Fund Product List." https://www.paho.org/sites/default/files/strategic-fund-product-list-230821_0.pdf.

Palomino, Sally. 2023. "El primer día como soldadas del Ejército de Colombia." *El País*, February 18, 2023, sec. América Colombia. https://elpais.com/america-colombia/2023-02-18/el-primer-dia-como-soldadas-del-ejercito-de-colombia.html.

Pardo, Raúl H., Olga Lucía Cabrera, Jorge Becerra, Patricia Fuya, and Cristina Ferro. 2006. "Lutzomyia longiflocosa as Suspected Vector of Cutaneous Leishmaniasis in a Focus of Cutaneous Leishmaniasis on the Sub-Andean Region of Tolima Department, Colombia, and the Knowledge on Sandflies by the Inhabitants." *Biomédica* 26 (October): 95–108. https://doi.org/10.7705/biomedica.v26i1.1504.

Parker, Melissa, and Tim Allen. 2014. "De-Politicizing Parasites: Reflections on Attempts to Control the Control of Neglected Tropical Diseases." *Medical Anthropology* 33 (3): 223–39. https://doi.org/10.1080/01459740.2013.831414.

Parker, Melissa, Hayley MacGregor, and Grace Akello. 2020. "COVID-19, Public Authority and Enforcement." *Medical Anthropology* 39 (8): 1–5. https://doi.org/10.1080/01459740.2020.1822833.

Parker, Richard, and Peter Aggleton. 2003. "HIV and AIDS-Related Stigma and Discrimination: A Conceptual Framework and Implications for Action." *Social Science & Medicine* 57 (1): 13–24.

Patino, Luz H., Claudia Mendez, Omaira Rodriguez, Yanira Romero, Daniel Velandia, Maria Alvarado, Julie Pérez, Maria Clara Duque, and Juan David Ramírez. 2017. "Spatial Distribution, Leishmania Species and Clinical Traits of Cutaneous Leishmaniasis Cases in the Colombian Army." *PLOS Neglected Tropical Diseases* 11 (8).

Pavli, Androula, and Helena C. Maltezou. 2010. "Leishmaniasis, an Emerging Infection in Travelers." *International Journal of Infectious Diseases* 14 (12): e1032–39.

PECET. 2015. "Leishmaniasis." Programa de Estudio y Control de Enfermedades Tropicales. 2015. http://www.pecet-colombia.org/site/leishmaniasis-enfermedad.html.

PECET and Fuerzas Militares de Colombia. 2005. *Enfermedades Tropicales: Guía de Manejo de ETV y Accidente Ofídico*. Medellín: PECET.

Pedersen, Duncan. 2002. "Political Violence, Ethnic Conflict, and Contemporary Wars: Broad Implications for Health and Social Well-Being." *Social Science & Medicine* 55 (2): 175–90.

Peluso, Nancy Lee, and Michael Watts, eds. 2001. *Violent Environments*. Ithaca, NY: Cornell University Press.

Pérez, Luis Eladio. 2008. *Infierno Verde: Siete Años Secuestrado por las FARC*. Madrid: Aguilar.

Perez-Franco, Jairo E., Mónica L. Cruz-Barrera, Marta L. Robayo, Myriam C. Lopez, Carlos D. Daza, Angela Bedoya, Maria L. Mariño, Carlos H. Saavedra, and Maria C. Echeverry. 2016. "Clinical and Parasitological Features of Patients with American Cutaneous Leishmaniasis That Did Not Respond to Treatment with Meglumine Antimoniate." *PLoS Neglected Tropical Diseases* 10 (5): e0004739. https://doi.org/10.1371/journal.pntd.0004739.

Perry, Heather R. 2014. *Recycling the Disabled: Army, Medicine, and Modernity in WWI Germany*. Manchester: Manchester University Press.

Petryna, Adriana. 2004. "Biological Citizenship: The Science and Politics of Chernobyl-Exposed Populations." *Osiris* 19:250–65.

Pinto-García, Lina. 2016. "Brote Epidémico de Leishmaniasis En Tolima." *El Espectador*, November 24, 2016. http://www.elespectador.com/noticias/salud/brote-epidemico-de-leishmaniasis-tolima-articulo-667147.

———. 2022. "Poisonously Single-Minded: Public Health Implications of the Pharmaceuticalization of Leishmaniasis in Colombia." *Critical Public Health* 32 (5): 619–29. https://doi.org/10.1080/09581596.2021.1918640.

———. 2023. "Addressing Two Rural Health Problems at Once: A Syndemic Approach to Malaria and Cutaneous Leishmaniasis in Post-Conflict Colombia." Institute for Science, Innovation & Society, University of Oxford.

———. 2025. "Unnecessary Adversaries Amidst War: Biomedical and Non-Biomedical Approaches to Leishmaniasis in Rural Colombia." In *Rural Disease Knowledge: Anthropological and Historical Perspectives*, edited by Matheus Alves Duarte da Silva and Christos Lynteris, 200–222. Abingdon: Routledge.

Platarrueda Vanegas, Claudia Patricia. 2008. "Contagio, Curación y Eficacia Terapéutica: Disensos Entre El Conocimiento Biomédico y El Conocimiento Vivencial de La Lepra En Colombia." *Antípoda*, no. 6, 171–95.

Pollock, Anne. 2011. "Transforming the Critique of Big Pharma." *BioSocieties* 6 (1): 106–18.

Profounda, Inc. 2023. "Leishmaniasis in the Military." Impavido. https://www.impavido.com/military.

Prosser, Jay. 2001. "Skin Memories." In *Thinking Through the Skin*, edited by Sara Ahmed and Jackie Stacey, 52–68. New York: Routledge.

Puar, Jasbir K. 2017. *The Right to Maim: Debility, Capacity, Disability*. Durham, NC: Duke University Press.

Pugliese, Joseph. 2020. *Biopolitics of the More-Than-Human: Forensic Ecologies of Violence*. Durham, NC: Duke University Press.

Quesada, James. 1998. "Suffering Child: An Embodiment of War and Its Aftermath in Post-Sandinista Nicaragua." *Medical Anthropology Quarterly* 12 (1): 51–73.

Quevedo, Emilio, Catalina Borda, Juan Carlos Eslava, Claudia Mónica García, María del Pilar Guzmán, Paola Mejía, and Carlos Noguera. 2004. *Café y gusanos, mosquitos y petróleo: El transito desde la higiene hacia la medicina tropical y la salud pública en Colombia, 1873–1953*. Bogotá: Universidad Nacional de Colombia.

Quevedo V., Emilio, Claudia Mónica García L., Joanna Bedoya D., Lisa Priscila Bustos J., Alain Camacho P., Carolina Manosalva R., Giovanna Matiz, Elquin Morales L., Juliana Pérez G., and Mónica Tafur A. 2017. *De Los Litorales a Las Selvas. La Construcción Del Concepto de Fiebre Amarilla, 1881–1938*. Bogotá: Universidad del Rosario. https://doi.org/10.12804/th9789587389029.

Quintero, Jorge. 2005. "Se duplicaron reportes de leishmaniasis en Caquetá." *El Tiempo*, December 7, 2005. https://www.eltiempo.com/archivo/documento/MAM-1853426.

Quintero, Viviana. 2009. "Huellas de las mismas botas." *El Espectador*, January 3, 2009. https://www.elespectador.com/opinion/huellas-de-las-mismas-botas-columna-103932.

Ramírez, María Clemencia. 2011. *Between the Guerrillas and the State: The Cocalero Movement, Citizenship, and Identity in the Colombian Amazon*. Durham, NC: Duke University Press.

Rath, Susanne, Luciano Augusto Trivelin, Talitha Rebecca Imbrunito, Daniela Maria Tomazela, Marcelo Nunes de Jesús, Percy Calvo Marzal, H. F. de Andrade, and André Gustavo Tempone. 2003. "Antimoniais Empregados No Tratamento Da Leishmaniose: Estado Da Arte." *Química Nova* 26 (4): 550–55.

Ravina, Enrique. 2011. *The Evolution of Drug Discovery: From Traditional Medicines to Modern Drugs*. John Wiley & Sons.

RCN. 2014. "Universidades no podrán exigir libreta militar para graduar estudiantes." Noticias RCN. December 2, 2014. https://noticias.canalrcn.com/nacional-pais/universidades-no-podran-exigir-libreta-militar-graduar-estudiantes.

RCN Radio. 2015. "Capturan en Bogotá a dos guerrilleros que almacenaban medicamentos." *RCN Radio*, September 8, 2015. https://www.rcnradio.com/colombia/capturan-en-bogota-a-dos-guerrilleros-que-almacenaban-medicamentos.

Redfield, Peter, and Edward B. Rackley. 2009. "Reintegration, or the Explosive Remnants of War." In *Catastrophe: Law, Politics, and the Humanitarian Impulse*, edited by Austin Sarat and Javier Lezaun. Amherst: University of Massachusetts Press.

Renne, Elisha P. 2014. "Parallel Dilemmas: Polio Transmission and Political Violence in Northern Nigeria." *Africa* 84 (3): 466–86. https://doi.org/10.1017/S0001972014000369.

Rheinberger, Hans-Joerg. 2000. "Beyond Nature and Culture: Modes of Reasoning in the Age of Molecular Biology and Medicine." In *Living and Working with the New Medical Technologies: Intersections of Inquiry*, edited by Margaret Lock, Allan Young, and Alberto Cambrosio, 19–30. Cambridge: Cambridge University Press.

Rico Mendoza, Andrea. 2016. "Seguridad Democrática, otro acierto del Plan Colombia en Boyacá." *El Tiempo*, February 4, 2016. https://www.eltiempo.com/archivo/documento/CMS-16500634.

RICYT. 2020. "El Estado de La Ciencia: Principales Indicadores de Ciencia y Tecnología Iberoamericanos / Interamericanos." http://www.ricyt.org/wp-content/uploads/2020/11/El EstadoDeLaCiencia_2020.pdf.

Rodríguez, Ileana. 1997. "Naturaleza/Nacion: Lo Salvaje/Civil Escribiendo Amazonia." *Revista de Crítica Literaria Latinoamericana* 23 (45): 27–42. https://doi.org/10.2307/4530889.

Rodríguez, Johana. 2020. "Corte aclara el tiempo de prestación del servicio militar obligatorio en Colombia." *RCN Radio*, February 27, 2020. https://www.rcnradio.com/judicial/corte-aclara-el-tiempo-de-prestacion-del-servicio-militar-obligatorio-en-colombia.

Rodríguez-Barraquer, Isabel, Rafael Góngora, Martín Prager, Robinson Pacheco, Luz Mery Montero, Adriana Navas, Cristina Ferro, Maria Consuelo Miranda, and Nancy G. Saravia. 2008. "Etiologic Agent of an Epidemic of Cutaneous Leishmaniasis in Tolima, Colombia." *American Journal of Tropical Medicine and Hygiene* 78 (2): 276–82. https://doi.org/10.4269/ajtmh.2008.78.276.

Rojas, Ricardo, Liliana Valderrama, Mabel Valderrama, Maria X. Varona, Marc Ouellette, and Nancy G. Saravia. 2006. "Resistance to Antimony and Treatment Failure in Human Leishmania (Viannia) Infection." *Journal of Infectious Diseases* 193 (10): 1375–83.

Rosales-Chilama, Mariana, Rafael E. Gongora, Liliana Valderrama, Jimena Jojoa, Neal Alexander, Luisa C. Rubiano, Alexandra Cossio, Emily R. Adams, Nancy G. Saravia, and María Adelaida Gomez. 2015. "Parasitological Confirmation and Analysis of *Leishmania* Diversity in Asymptomatic and Subclinical Infection Following Resolution of Cutaneous

Leishmaniasis." *PLoS Neglected Tropical Diseases* 9 (12). https://doi.org/10.1371/journal.pntd.0004273.

Rose, Nikolas, and Carlos Novas. 2005. "Biological Citizenship." In *Global Assemblages: Technology, Politics, and Ethics as Anthropological Problems*, edited by Aihwa Ong and Stephen J. Collier, 439–63. Malden, MA: Blackwell.

Ruiz-Serna, Daniel. 2023. *When Forests Run Amok: War and Its Afterlives in Indigenous and Afro-Colombian Territories*. Durham, NC: Duke University Press.

Ruiz-Serna, Daniel, and Diana Ojeda. 2023. *Belicopedia*. Bogotá: Universidad de los Andes.

Ruta Pacífica de las Mujeres. 2013. "La Verdad de Las Mujeres En El Conflicto Armado En Colombia, Tomo II." http://rutapacifica.org.co/documentos/tomo-II.pdf.

Santaella, Julián, Clara B. Ocampo, Nancy G. Saravia, Fabián Méndez, Rafael Góngora, Maria Adelaida Gomez, Leonard E. Munstermann, and Rupert J. Quinnell. 2011. "*Leishmania* (*Viannia*) Infection in the Domestic Dog in Chaparral, Colombia." *American Journal of Tropical Medicine and Hygiene* 84 (5): 674–80. https://doi.org/10.4269/ajtmh.2011.10-0159.

Saravia, Nancy Gore, and Rubén Santiago Nicholls. 2006. "Leishmaniasis: Un Reto Para La Salud Pública Que Exige Concertación de Voluntades y Esfuerzos." *Biomédica* 26 (1): 5–9.

Seaman, J., A. J. Mercer, and E. Sondorp. 1996. "The Epidemic of Visceral Leishmaniasis in Western Upper Nile, Southern Sudan: Course and Impact from 1984 to 1994." *International Journal of Epidemiology* 25 (4): 862–71.

Seaman, Rebecca, ed. 2018. *Epidemics and War: The Impact of Disease on Major Conflicts in History*. Santa Barbara, CA: ABC-CLIO.

Segal, Naomi. 2009. *Consensuality: Didier Anzieu, Gender and the Sense of Touch*. Amsterdam: Brill.

Semana. 2015. "Reveladores audios de cómo extorsionan a los colombianos desde las cárceles." *Semana*, August 15, 2015. https://www.semana.com/nacion/articulo/extorsiones-desde-prisiones-van-en-aumento/438639-3.

———. 2017. "La última marcha de las Farc." *Semana*, February 4, 2017. https://www.semana.com/nacion/articulo/farc--se-concentraron-en-zonas-veredales/514346.

———. n.d. "La bolsa o la vida." La bolsa o la vida, Sección Nación, edición 1500, Jan 29 2011. Accessed April 27, 2018. https://www.semana.com/nacion/articulo/la-bolsa-vida/234832-3.

Serje, Margarita. 2005. *El revés de la nación: Territorios salvajes, fronteras y tierras de nadie*. Bogotá: Universidad de los Andes.

———. 2014. "La Selva Por Cárcel." In *El Paraíso Del Diablo: Roger Casement y El Informe Del Putumayo*, edited by C. Steiner, C. Páramo, and R. Rineda Camacho, 151–71. Bogotá: Universidad de los Andes, Universidad Nacional de Colombia.

Serrano, Sebastián. 2017. "Traté de sacar mi libreta militar con la nueva ley (y no es tan fácil como creía)." *¡PACIFISTA!* (blog). September 13, 2017. https://pacifista.tv/notas/trate-de-sacar-mi-libreta-militar-con-la-nueva-ley-y-no-es-tan-facil-como-creia/.

Serrano-Amaya, Jose Fernando. 2013. "A People-Centered Approach to the Links among HIV/AIDS, Conflicts, and Security in Colombia." In *Global HIV/AIDS Politics, Policy, and Activism: Persistent Challenges and Emerging Issues*, edited by Raymond A. Smith, 1:315–35. Santa Barbara, CA: Praeger.

Sharara, Sima L., and Souha S. Kanj. 2014. "War and Infectious Diseases: Challenges of the Syrian Civil War." *PLoS Pathogens* 10 (11): e1004438.

Slater, Leo. 2009. *War and Disease: Biomedical Research on Malaria in the Twentieth Century*. New Brunswick, NJ: Rutgers University Press.

Smallman-Raynor, Matthew. 2004. *War Epidemics: An Historical Geography of Infectious Diseases in Military Conflict and Civil Strife, 1850–2000*. Oxford Geographical and Environmental Studies. Oxford: Oxford University Press.

Smart, Alan, and Filippo Zerilli. 2014. "Extralegality." In *A Companion to Urban Anthropology*, edited by Donald M. Nonini, 222–38. Malden, MA: Wiley Blackwell.

Stepan, Nancy Leys. 2015. *Eradication: Ridding the World of Diseases Forever?* Ithaca, NY: Cornell University Press.

Steverding, Dietmar. 2017. "The History of Leishmaniasis." *Parasites & Vectors* 10 (February): 82. https://doi.org/10.1186/s13071-017-2028-5.

Strathern, Marilyn. 1980. "No Nature, No Culture: The Hagen Case." In *Nature, Culture and Gender*, edited by Carol P. MacCormack and Marilyn Strathern, 174–222. Cambridge: Cambridge University Press.

Suchman, Lucy. 2015. "Situational Awareness: Deadly Bioconvergence at the Boundaries of Bodies and Machines." *MediaTropes* 5 (1): 1–24.

Sundar, Shyam, and Jaya Chakravarty. 2010. "Antimony Toxicity." *International Journal of Environmental Research and Public Health* 7 (12): 4267. https://doi.org/10.3390/ijerph7124267.

Tamayo-Agudelo, William, and Vaughan Bell. 2019. "Armed Conflict and Mental Health in Colombia." *BJPsych International* 16 (2): 40–42. https://doi.org/10.1192/bji.2018.4.

Taussig, Michael. 1999. *Defacement: Public Secrecy and the Labor of the Negative*. Stanford, CA: Stanford University Press.

Territorio Chocoano. 2011. "Decomisan En El Bajo Baudó Medicina Para La Leishmaniasis." *Territorio Chocoano*, August 29, 2011. http://www.territoriochocoano.com/secciones/orden-publico/1828-decomisan-en-el-bajo-baudo-medicina-para-la-leishmaniasis.html.

Terry, Jennifer. 2017. *Attachments to War: Biomedical Logics and Violence in Twenty-First-Century America*. Durham, NC: Duke University Press.

Thomson, Mathew. 1998. "Status, Manpower and Mental Fitness: Mental Deficiency in the First World War." In *War, Medicine and Modernity*, edited by Roger Cooter, Steve Sturdy, and Mark Harrison, 149–66. Stroud: Sutton.

Timmermans, Stefan, and Marc Berg. 2003. *The Gold Standard: The Challenge of Evidence-Based Medicine*. Philadelphia: Temple University Press.

Timmermans, Stefan, and Steven Epstein. 2010. "A World of Standards but Not a Standard World: Toward a Sociology of Standards and Standardization." *Annual Review of Sociology* 36 (1): 69–89.

Timmermans, Stefan, and Rebecca Kaufman. 2020. "Technologies and Health Inequities." *Annual Review of Sociology* 46 (1): 583–602. https://doi.org/10.1146/annurev-soc-121919-054802.

Tironi, Manuel. 2018. "Hypo-Interventions: Intimate Activism in Toxic Environments." *Social Studies of Science* 48 (3): 438–55. https://doi.org/10.1177/0306312718784779.

Tuon, Felipe Francisco, Valdir Sabbaga Amato, Maria Esther Graf, Andre Machado Siqueira, Antonio Carlos Nicodemo, and Vicente Amato Neto. 2008. "Treatment of New World Cutaneous Leishmaniasis—A Systematic Review with a Meta-Analysis." *International Journal of Dermatology* 47 (2): 109–24. https://doi.org/10.1111/j.1365-4632.2008.03417.x.

United Nations. 2023. "United Nations Verification Mission in Colombia—Report of the Secretary-General." https://colombia.unmissions.org/sites/default/files/n2317646_en.pdf.

Uribe de Hincapié, María Teresa. 2001. *Nación, Ciudadano y Soberano*. Medellín: Corporación Región.

Urrego Mendoza, Diana Zulima. 2003. "Narrativas de Médicos Colombianos En Contexto de Guerra." Manizales: Universidad de Manizales.

Urrego Mendoza, Zulma. 2011. "De Protestas, Violencias y Otras Fiebres Tropicales: Aportes Para Una Historia Socio-Política de La Salud Pública En Colombia, 1974–2004." Bogotá: Universidad Nacional de Colombia. http://www.bdigital.unal.edu.co/4452/.

———. 2015. "Conflicto Armado En Colombia y Misión Médica: Narrativas de Médicos Como Memorias de Supervivencia." *Revista de La Facultad de Medicina* 63 (3): 377–88. https://doi.org/10.15446/revfacmed.v63n3.45209.

US Embassy in Colombia. 2005a. "Cable: 05BOGOTA3217_a." WikiLeaks. https://wikileaks.org/plusd/cables/05BOGOTA3217_a.html.

———. 2005b. "Cable: 05BOGOTA3937_a." WikiLeaks. https://wikileaks.org/plusd/cables/05BOGOTA3937_a.html.

———. 2005c. "Cable: 05BOGOTA8545_a." WikiLeaks. https://wikileaks.org/plusd/cables/05BOGOTA8545_a.html.

———. 2005d. "Cable: 05BOGOTA8696_a." WikiLeaks. https://wikileaks.org/plusd/cables/05BOGOTA8696_a.html.

———. 2006a. "Cable: 06BOGOTA1369_a." WikiLeaks. https://wikileaks.org/plusd/cables/06BOGOTA1369_a.html.

———. 2006b. "Cable: 06BOGOTA11382_a." WikiLeaks. https://wikileaks.org/plusd/cables/06BOGOTA11382_a.html.

Vacca, Claudia, José Orozco, Albert Figueras, and Dolors Capellà. 2005. "Assessment of Risks Related to Medicine Dispensing by Nonprofessionals in Colombia: Clinical Case Simulations." *Annals of Pharmacotherapy* 39 (3): 527–32. https://doi.org/10.1345/aph.1E420.

Vacca, Claudia, Claudia Yaneth Niño, and Ludovic Reveiz. 2011. "Restricción de la venta de antibióticos en farmacias de Bogotá, Colombia: Estudio descriptivo." *Revista Panamericana de Salud Pública* 30 (December): 586–91. https://doi.org/10.1590/S1020-49892011001200015.

Valderrama-Ardila, Carlos, Neal Alexander, Cristina Ferro, Horacio Cadena, Dairo Marín, Theodore R. Holford, Leonard E. Munstermann, and Clara B. Ocampo. 2010. "Environmental Risk Factors for the Incidence of American Cutaneous Leishmaniasis in a Sub-Andean Zone of Colombia (Chaparral, Tolima)." *American Journal of Tropical Medicine and Hygiene* 82 (2): 243–50. https://doi.org/10.4269/ajtmh.2010.09-0218.

Valencia, Carlos Fernando, Jorge Andrés Suárez, Álvaro Cogollos, Ricardo Augusto Uribe, and Gloria Carmenza Flores. 2015. "Heridos en combate, experiencia del Grupo de Trauma del Hospital Militar Central de Bogotá." *Revista Colombiana de Cirugía* 30 (1). http://www.redalyc.org/resumen.oa?id=355538978005.

Valencia, León, and Carlos Montoya. 2016. "Las Bandas Criminales y el Postconflicto." *Blog Fundación Paz y Reconciliación* (blog). February 24, 2016. https://pares.com.co/2016/02/24/las-bandas-criminales-y-el-postconflicto/.

Van der Geest, Sjaak, Susan Reynolds Whyte, and Anita Hardon. 1996. "The Anthropology of Pharmaceuticals: A Biographical Approach." *Annual Review of Anthropology*, 153–78.

Vanderslott, Samantha. 2019. "Moving from Outsider to Insider Status through Metrics: The Inclusion of 'Neglected Tropical Diseases' into the Sustainable Development Goals." *Journal of Human Development and Capabilities* 20 (4): 418–35. https://doi.org/10.1080/19452829.2019.1574727.

Vanguardia. 2014. "Ejército incautó encomienda con un medicamento contra la leshmaniasis." *Vanguardia*, April 28, 2014. https://www.vanguardia.com/judicial/ejercito-incauto-encomienda-con-un-medicamento-contra-la-leshmaniasis-KEVL257379.

Vega, Juan Carlos, Boris Fernando Sanchez, Luz Mery Montero, Rafael Montaña, Mercedes Del Pilar Mahecha, Bladimir Dueñes, Angela Rocío Baron, and Richard Reithinger. 2007. "Short Communication: The Cost-Effectiveness of Cutaneous Leishmaniasis Patient Management during an Epidemic in Chaparral, Colombia in 2004." *Tropical Medicine & International Health: TM & IH* 12 (12): 1540–44. https://doi.org/10.1111/j.1365-3156.2007.01962.x.

———. 2009. "The Efficacy of Thermotherapy to Treat Cutaneous Leishmaniasis in Colombia: A Comparative Observational Study in an Operational Setting." *Transactions of the Royal Society of Tropical Medicine and Hygiene* 103 (7): 703–6. https://doi.org/10.1016/j.trstmh.2008.10.039.

Vélez, Iván Darío, Erik Hendrickx, Sara María Robledo, and Sonia del Pilar Agudelo. 2001. "Leishmaniosis Cutánea En Colombia y Género." *Cadernos de Saúde Pública* 17 (1): 171–80. https://doi.org/10.1590/S0102-311X2001000100018.

Vélez, Juanita, and Juan Pablo Pérez. 2016. "Leishmaniasis, La Enfermedad Del Posconflicto." *La Silla Vacía*, December 8, 2016. http://lasillavacia.com/historia/leishmaniasis-la-enfermedad-del-posconflicto-59023.

Verdad Abierta. 2009a. "Carlos Tijeras reconoce asesinato de joven colombo francés." *Verdad Abierta* (blog), September 2, 2009. https://verdadabierta.com/carlos-tijeras-reconoce-asesinato-de-joven-colombo-frances/.

———. 2009b. "Trámite de la Ley de Justicia y Paz, Audiencia de Formulación de Imputación contra John Esquivel Cuadrado." *Verdad Abierta* (blog). Accessed July 13, 2015. http://www.verdadabierta.com/listado-imputaciones/john-esquivel-cuadrado-alias-el-tigre/87-audiencia-de-imputacion-del-07112008-1/file&sa=U&ei=rgC_U6qlN4GayATG0oGwDg&ved=0CA8QFjAG&client=internal-uds-cse&usg=AFQjCNGuc1NfcifBW5.

———. 2010. "Imputan 13 masacres y 491 desplazamientos a 'El Tigre.'" *Verdad Abierta* (blog), January 22, 2010. https://verdadabierta.com/imputan-13-masacres-y-491-desplazamientos-a-el-tigre/.

———. 2011. "Condenan a 'Carlos Tijeras' por asesinato de colombo-francés." *Verdad Abierta* (blog). June 13, 2011. https://verdadabierta.com/condenan-a-carlos-tijeras-por-asesinato-de-colombo-frances/.

———. 2013. "Así se formó el Bloque Oriental de las Farc." *Verdad Abierta* (blog), March 11, 2013. https://verdadabierta.com/asi-se-formo-el-bloque-oriental-de-las-farc/.

———. 2017. "Pese a no estar listas las zonas, Farc pueden concentrarse." *Verdad Abierta* (blog), January 26, 2017. https://verdadabierta.com/pese-a-no-estar-listas-farc-pueden-concentrarse-en-zonas-veredales/.

Vergel, Carolina, Ricardo Palacios, Horacio Cadena, Claudia Jimena Posso, Liliana Valderrama, Mauricio Perez, John Walker, Bruno Luis Travi, and Nancy Gore Saravia. 2006. "Evidence for Leishmania (Viannia) Parasites in the Skin and Blood of Patients before and after Treatment." *Journal of Infectious Diseases* 194 (4): 503–11. https://doi.org/10.1086/505583.

Vianna, Gaspar. 1912. "Tratamento Da Leishmaniose Tegumentar Por Injeções Intravenosas de Tártaro Emético." In *Anais Do 7o Congresso Brasileiro de Medicina e Cirurgia*, 426–28.

Vincent, H. M. 2017. "William Boog Leishman: Parasitologist and Politician." *Parasitology* 144 (12): 1582–89. https://doi.org/10.1017/S0031182016001657.

Wasserstein, Ronald L., Allen L. Schirm, and Nicole A. Lazar. 2019. "Moving to a World Beyond 'p < 0.05.'" *American Statistician* 73 (Suppl. 1): 1–19. https://doi.org/10.1080/00031305.2019.1583913.

Weigle, Kristen A., Cecilia Santrich, Fernando Martinez, Liliana Valderrama, and Nancy G. Saravia. 1993. "Epidemiology of Cutaneous Leishmaniasis in Colombia: Environmental and Behavioral Risk Factors for Infection, Clinical Manifestations, and Pathogenicity." *Journal of Infectious Diseases* 168 (3): 709–14.

Westerhaus, Michael. 2007. "Linking Anthropological Analysis and Epidemiological Evidence: Formulating a Narrative of HIV Transmission in Acholiland of Northern Uganda." *SAHARA-J* 4 (2): 590–605.

Whitmarsh, Ian. 2008. "Biomedical Ambivalence: Asthma Diagnosis, the Pharmaceutical, and Other Contradictions in Barbados." *American Ethnologist* 35 (1): 49–63. https://doi.org/10.1111/j.1548-1425.2008.00005.x.

WHO. 2009. "Frequently Asked Questions about the International Health Regulations (2005)." https://www.who.int/ihr/about/FAQ2009.pdf.

———. 2010. "Control of the Leishmaniases: Report of a Meeting of the WHO Expert Committee on the Control of Leishmaniases, Geneva, 22–26 March 2010." 949. WHO Technical Report Series. Geneva: WHO.

———. n.d. "Neglected Tropical Diseases." WHO. Accessed May 7, 2019. http://www.who.int/neglected_diseases/diseases/en/.

Wickham-Crowley, Timothy P. 1992. *Guerrillas and Revolution in Latin America: A Comparative Study of Insurgents and Regimes since 1956*. Princeton, NJ: Princeton University Press.

Widger, Tom. 2018. "Suicides, Poisons and the Materially Possible: The Positive Ambivalence of Means Restriction and Critical–Critical Global Health." *Journal of Material Culture* 23 (4): 396–412. https://doi.org/10.1177/1359183518799525.

Wieringa, Sietse, Eivind Engebretsen, Kristin Heggen, and Trish Greenhalgh. 2017. "Has Evidence-Based Medicine Ever Been Modern? A Latour-Inspired Understanding of a Changing EBM." *Journal of Evaluation in Clinical Practice* 23 (5): 964–70. https://doi.org/10.1111/jep.12752.

Williams, Simon, Paul Martin, and Jonathan Gabe. 2011. "The Pharmaceuticalisation of Society? A Framework for Analysis." *Sociology of Health & Illness* 33 (5): 710–25. https://doi.org/10.1111/j.1467-9566.2011.01320.x.

Winegard, Timothy C. 2019. *The Mosquito: A Human History of Our Deadliest Predator*. New York: Dutton.

Woodhouse, Edward, David Hess, Steve Breyman, and Brian Martin. 2002. "Science Studies and Activism: Possibilities and Problems for Reconstructivist Agendas." *Social Studies of Science* 32 (2): 297–319.

Wool, Zoë H. 2015. *After War: The Weight of Life at Walter Reed*. Durham, NC: Duke University Press.

Worboys, Michael. 2003. "Colonial Medicine." In *Companion to Medicine in the Twentieth Century*, edited by Roger Cooter and John Pickstone, 1st ed. London: Routledge.

Wortmann, Glenn, R. Scott Miller, Charles Oster, Joan Jackson, and Naomi Aronson. 2002. "A Randomized, Double-Blind Study of the Efficacy of a 10-or 20-Day Course of Sodium

Stibogluconate for Treatment of Cutaneous Leishmaniasis in United States Military Personnel." *Clinical Infectious Diseases* 35 (3): 261–67.

Zamudio Palma, Mario. 2017. "Policarpa, la zona veredal que ya no fue." *Pacifista*, May 12, 2017. http://pacifista.co/policarpa-la-zona-veredal-que-ya-no-fue/.

Zapor, Michael J., and Kimberly A. Moran. 2005. "Infectious Diseases during Wartime." *Current Opinion in Infectious Diseases* 18:395–99.

Zinsser, Hans. 2010. *Rats, Lice and History*. New Brunswick: Transaction.

Zola, Irving Kenneth. 1972. "Medicine as an Institution of Social Control." *Sociological Review* 20 (4): 487–504. https://doi.org/10.1111/j.1467-954X.1972.tb00220.x.

Zuleta, Monica, and Iván Darío Vélez. 2014. "Geografía de La Expansión de La Leishmaniasis En El Conflicto Armado En Colombia (Antioquia)." *EU-Topías* 7. http://eu-topias.org/articulo.php?ref_page=501.

Index

The letter *f* following a page number denotes a figure.